THE
MYTHOLOGY
of
CATS

Feline Legend and Lore through the Ages

THE
MYTHOLOGY
of
CATS

Gerald and Loretta Hausman

BERKLEY BOOKS, NEW YORK

THE MYTHOLOGY OF CATS

"Nansen" by Gary Snyder is gratefully reprinted from *No Nature: New and Selected Poems*, published by New Directions Publishing Corporation.

"Pangur Ban" is reprinted with thanks to the Storytellers of Sanibel, Noel and Bert McCarry.

"The Cat" by David Kherdian is gratefully reprinted from *Threads of Light*, published by Two Rivers Press.

A Berkley Book / published by arrangement with
St. Martin's Press, LLC.

PRINTING HISTORY
St. Martin's Press hardcover edition / August 1998
Berkley trade paperback edition / August 2000

The Penguin Putnam Inc. World Wide Web site address is
http://www.penguinputnam.com

ISBN: 0-425-17449-2

BERKLEY®
Berkley Books are published by The Berkley Publishing Group,
a division of Penguin Putnam Inc.,
375 Hudson Street, New York, New York 10014.
BERKLEY and the "B" design are trademarks
belonging to Penguin Putnam Inc.

PRINTED IN THE UNITED STATES OF AMERICA

10 9 8 7 6 5 4 3 2 1

Contents

Acknowledgments

W E WISH TO thank the following individuals who were invaluable in helping us with this book: Mariah Fox Hausman, illustrator, Cutler Ridge, Florida; Hannah Hausman, researcher at the Richter Library of the University of Miami, Coral Gables, Flordia; Philippe Brian Greaux, author, Coral Gables, Flordia; Jane Lindskold, author, Albuquerque, New Mexico. We are also grateful for the Internet cat correspondents who furnished us with piquant and relevant tales: Virginia Andrews, Geoff Lalagy, J. Symmons-Brown. Special thanks to cat owners Janette Healy and Joanne Merritt, both of Pine Island, Flordia; and Miriam and Mitzi of Deer Isle, Maine. Lastly, a tip of the whisker to Sanibel Storytellers, Noel and Bert McCarry, for their faithful cat lore and encouragement; and to Bob Weil of St. Martin's, whose love of animals brought us all together again.

Introduction: The Archetypal Cat

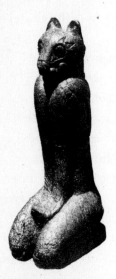

Calusa cat motif

Going back to the ancient Egyptian sun priests, we find that the archetypal cat was a sun god and moon goddess, each a deity of fecundity. Cats blessed weddings and births, and were always present at deaths, as they carried human spirits from this world to the next. Cats were connected to the cosmos as no other animal, and because of this they granted us our own vestigial link to the spheres and the powers thereof that gave us spiritual strength.

The archetypal cat is still with us, mysteriously alive in the collective unconscious. But how did the mythos of Felidae, beginning, some say, in 1590 B.C.E., spread worldwide—so pervasively as to reach all the way into the cusp of the twenty-first century?

In answer, we may refer to one cat myth that sped across the centuries, traveling from the desert sand of ancient Egypt to the heathered hills of Scotland. It seems that when the Greek general Galsthelos was defeated by the miracle of the Red Sea parting before his armies, he fled. With him was his wife, Scota, Pharaoh's daughter, who brought her cats with her. In memory of this beautiful woman the country of Scotland was named when a descendant of Galsthelos, Fergus I, became the ruler of that kingdom. And the mascot cats that Scota brought out of Egypt thus became the symbols, the archetypes, the myths of yet another land, the two coming together in spiritual union.

This is but one example of how archetypes are founded and generated and buried deeply, and subtly, in the human psyche. What we seem to remember from our ancient past glitters in the imagery of the present. The old ways, as preserved in mythology, take us to places where we have roved and rambled only in dream. And yet, such intimations that burn in our blood are no less real for being imaginary. We have only to look into the common house cat's moony eye to feel the presence of shadows and twilights beyond the reach of time.

The archetypal cat is an animal more spiritual than natural— thus, supernatural. From the earliest of times, we have looked to cats for religious guidance. Accordingly, we have given them roles of leadership that would elevate us with them, and, hopefully, put us on the same etheric plane, as equals.

The myths themselves counsel us in everyday morals and manners. These are the tales of the talking cat, the angel cat, the healing cat, the traveling cat, the psychic cat, the immortal cat, the working cat, the mother cat, the artistic cat, to name just a few. All cultures have such mundane, yet mystical cats, and they are role models of a very positive kind, unlike the more popular archetypes of disaster, demonology, darkness, and depravity. For though these are also founded in mythology, we believe they are demeaning and do not bear further publication. Our preference is for the *matagot,* the French good luck cat, as opposed to the devil's familiar, the negative witch cat.

After exploring each myth archetypally, we have added a page or two of breed information, qualifying rather than quantifying the cat to whom the myth appears to be connected. The bobtail legends of the Isle of Man go back to tales of the ark, but the cat, in this instance, is the Manx, and can really be no other. We have included more than twenty known breeds, but only where they lent themselves naturally, rather than artificially, to the given mythology.

Cats cannot really be known in a book—we must experience them to know them. And yet mythology brings us to a different kind of cat experience—that of another time, another place, another world. In so knowing the cat, we may know ourselves—anew. The ancient Egyptians worshiped the feline and wrought a complex mythology around her that included the serpent, the raptor, the human being. The cat goddess could speak in many tongues, see through many eyes, and walk on winged feet. She still does. Look into her eyes.

GERALD AND LORETTA HAUSMAN

THE GODDESS CAT

Egyptian Mau

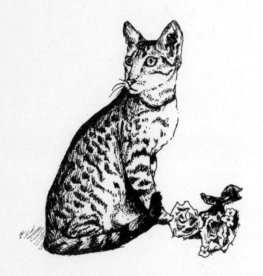

T HE CAT, A creature of light and dark in Egyptian mythology, is lion-headed and moon-eyed, a feline, born of duality. Indeed, the cat in ancient times appeared male in one incarnation and female in another. The sun god, Ra, was male, but the goddess of femininity and maternity, Bastet, or Bast, was female.

It was Bastet who had the body of a woman and the head of a cat, an image that down the centuries has produced a cornucopia of cat mythology. Arguably, our modern notion of cats as being female (dogs are male) comes from the allegorical tradition that sprang up along the eastern branch of the Nile and the town known as Bubastis.

Bastet was a pervasive figure in Egypt from about 2000 B.C.E. Princes, priests, and common people alike revered her, and her image was seen in murals and burials and gazing down from immense effigies that shadowed the Nile. As cat historian Fernand Mery explains, "The goddess was a disturbing creature whom every Egyptian woman wished to resemble in the strangeness of her gaze, her slanting eyes, her supple loins, her noble posture and her animal abandon."

This *femina* and *felis* relationship is given sanctimony in a poem by fourteen-year-old poet Cathy Thomas:

> *Ah, Cat, you are Woman,*
> *You are the first and the last breath of love;*
> *You filter off my red today.*
> *You were sacred when the Walls fell down,*
> *Now scarred you remain*
> *The survivor of a barren earth,*
> *A void sky.*
> *Like woman, you arise;*
> *Like woman, you take your bed*
> *Among the stars.*

In this little poem, we see the woman as a cat goddess; the cat as a victim of genocide. We are told that the cat is a survivor and the denizen of the heavenly bodies. We see the cat of persecutions, sitting on a silky cushion, purring a song to the Milky Way.

Among the many known attributes of cats, there is one that it shares with the human female. We are referring to the misnamed quotient called "woman's intuition." Cats and moons, cycles of lunar order and disorder, reign in the human imagination, but they always return to the matriarchal earth mother religions of our ancestors. These were people who believed, like the Native Americans, that the sun was the father and the earth was the mother.

The mother's aspect is always one of adoration, adoption, protection. Seeing into the future has, since the dynasty that produced the Colossi of Memnon, been the province of women. Nor is this restricted to the ancient Egyptian culture, for the classic kimono cat of Japan is female. So is Freya, cat goddess of Helle, queen of the Nordic underworld. The cleanliness of the cat, so treasured by the

Muslims, was feminine, sequestered, and removed from the jurisdiction of men.

However, there is no getting around the pervasive feminine mystique of the cat as fostered by the the Egyptian dynasties. An interesting sidelight is how the first cats came to Scotland, and it explains why the cat there has a female nobility. Beginning on the banks of the Nile, the Greek general Galsthelos, who commanded Pharaoh's army, was defeated at the parting of the waters of the Red Sea. Galsthelos lived to see another day, though, and traveled with his wife, Scota, who was the Pharaoh's daughter. Eventually, the general came to Portugal and settled there, but some centuries later, his descendant founded a country far to the north, and he named it after his ancestress, the beautiful Scota. That country he called Scotland and its mascot was a cat, a relative of the Egyptian Mau.

One reason why cats have been given female nomenclature in modern times is that the behavior of the cat has always been, and continues to be, puzzling—especially to men. Statistically, American men still prefer dogs over cats.

The author Claude Farrere once described an occurrence wherein his cat "leapt backwards and spun round wildly, his tail absolutely stiff. He tried to fly." Here was a normal cat suddenly subjected to a thousand sensations of madness. It took a long time, Farrere said, for his pet to finally calm down. The following day, the author discovered that at exactly the same moment that his cat tried to soar through the air, the young woman next door took her life.

One might conclude that, at any given time, cats know much more than we do. For they can visualize what we cannot. Another way of saying this is that only half the story is ever told, and that, of course is the human half. If the cat's side of the saga were told it might reveal quite a lot about us humans.

Sylvia Townsend Warner gives us a tantalizing clue in her tale "The Traveller from the West and the Traveller from the East."

The first half of it is about a forlorn man, whose wife has cat's blood, and though she is extremely attractive, she likes to eat mice in bed, and to stare vacantly at the moon. This is an old European myth that stems from an older Egyptian one. Yet, there is the other half of the story—the cat's cradle of feline misfortune.

It seems that a certain cat, having come to the house of a widow woman, decides to provide for her. The woman, seeing the cat's industry as a poulterer, says that he is indeed a true cat and kinder than any man. In all kinds of weather, then, and dodging farmers' bullets and trappers' nets, the cat captures and kills hens, ducks, pigeons, wild fowl, rabbits, and hares. And the widow sells them out of her house. But as time goes on, her love of money overcomes her good sense, and she sets her prices so high that no one can afford to buy her meats.

In the end, they rot and they stink, and the whole house reeks.

Now the cat despairs over his affair with the widow, for there is nothing so loathsome to a cat than an ill-smelling house. As the cat says, "How could it be a pleasure to love a person so obviously lazy, greedy, dirty, and inefficient? I was forced to admit it: she was no more than human."

When the cat leaves the tavern where he's told this sad, sad tale, the wind rises in the trees and lightning flickers in the forest, and the talk, once again, turns to ghosts, famine, poverty, and pestilence.

And that, it seems, sums up the human condition. No wonder the goddess cat, with golden eyes turned inward, longs for the palmy days and desert nights, where sweet incense burned at her feet, and where the punishment for violating her was the sentence of death.

The Lore of the Cat

The Egyptian Mau is a quintessential figure of all that was, and all that is, catlike. She was there at the beginning, listening to the whispers of the worshipers in the marbled halls of Bubastis.

The Egyptian Mau seems to suggest all the old feline symbolism, and there is quite a lot of it—from the cat's eye being lunar, filling to fullness and then dimming, to the conflict of the cat sun, Ra, and the snake moon, Apep—the two always in a contest to rule the domain of light or dark.

Oldest of known domestic cats, the Mau was depicted on scroll and temple wall in 1400 B.C.E.

The Mau's physical constitution, owing perhaps to its royal lineage, is susceptible to illness. Cold weather, sudden seasonal change—these are hard for her to bear. She is beautiful, and whether smoke, silver, bronze, or pewter, she is especially lovely to behold.

There is a noticeable scarab beetle pattern on the brows of this cat, as well as mascara lines on the cheeks. Random spots decorate the body, running to broken lines. The paws are egg-shaped. Antiquity has definitely left its mark on this cat's rare beauty. The almond eyes and large and long pointed ears combine to give the face a masquelike perfection, as if, although mummified, it had suddenly sprung to life.

The cat-and-serpent motif has been compared, in mythology, to the virgin and the dragon. As the virgin mother, the sacred cat of the Nile was sometimes invoked as Isis, as this famous female deity could also assume feline form. In this capacity, she became the slayer of serpents. This is why the Egyptians believed that the bite of an asp could be cured by a cat.

Atet was queen of the gods; her symbol, the cat. Lioness, perhaps. Cat nonetheless.

In later dynasties, the symbology changed. The new ruling deity was the golden male figure whose name was Ra. He personified the life-sustaining sun that vanquished the darkness and the dead, the shadow and the serpent. To accomplish these feats, Ra assumed the form of a cat. So the slayer of the serpent of darkness now became a male deity, but he possessed many of the female qualities exhibited by his predecessors, Atet and Isis.

When more millennia passed, the vague archetypes of the Egyptians turned into an unconscious memory. Perhaps a flash of these old images, stored in the brain forever, may remind us, may even tickle us, when we see the silky presence of a lovely cat. For here is a creature that encompasses a world order long gone, a mythical voyage into the vastness of space and time.

THE CARETAKER CAT

Russian Blue

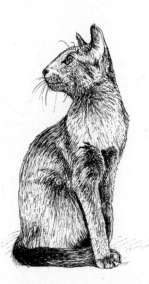

THE FOLKTALE OF the overdressed puss who swaggers his master's impoverishment into incalculable wealth is a truly universal fable. In fact, Carl Van Vechten author of *The Tiger in the House,* claims that every country on earth where there are cats has a caretaker cat myth, and while these may differ in details, in the main, they are the same.

The plot is generally that a cat comes to help someone. In gaining the person's trust, the cat's spirit somehow manifests either riches or rewards—these can be spiritual, or material, or both. The allegory of the Puss in Boots fable is that the cat isn't really the benefactor, but rather the human being's trust of the cat is what turns misfortune into personal gain.

Contemporary animated films like Disney's *Aristocats,* as well as the saga of *Homeward Bound,* and even *That Darned Cat* all speak of cat caretakers; cats as charmers, healers, and helpmates in a world that would often do without them. In the real world, cats have never been in greater demand as companions to the elderly, the terminally ill, the afflicted.

Interestingly enough, the history of the caretaker cat seems to predate that of man's best friend, the dog. Egyptian alchemy notwithstanding, cat medicine and divination existed in the Holocene epoch, when panthers, leopards, and lynxes were first recognizable to our fire-crouching ancestors.

The efficiency of the great predator cats led us, as would-be hunters, into observing cat kills, and then noticing other, less visible, orders of cat power. These have been with us for ten thousand years, during which time we have used the cat, devotionally and medicinally. Patricia Dale-Green, author of *Cult of the Cat,* speaks about our primal relationship with the feline:

> In Scotland single standing stones of the Neolithic age are often known as "cat stanes"; and near Maidstone, in Kent, there is a famous cromlech, consisting of a vast block of sandstone resting on three other blocks, which is known as Kit's Coty House. No one knows why such ancient monuments should be associated with cats, but they are symbols of indestructibility and perpetuity.

The talismanic cat, whose power to heal is blessed by gods of unknown origin, is European rather than Egyptian. The Egyptians knew where the cat's power originated; we, evidently, have forgotten. Yet we still honor the cat that heals, and never before in human history have more people joined together to experience whatever it is that the cat has, does, or, as catalyst, causes to happen. Perhaps, as some cat experts say, our identification with the cat is enough to bring about self-healing; as we love the animal, we extend love to ourselves and outward to others around us. This in itself is a profound act of beneficence, one capable of engendering well-being. Helen Howard, a clinical psychologist, writing about a young woman addicted to amphetamines observed the change she saw in her patient when she adopted a Russian Blue.

The striking thing about the girl, whose name was Lana, and the cat, whose name was Greyman, was their acute similarity. Both of them were beautiful, graceful. Each had large green eyes set like gems in a wide-boned Slavic face that, despite the lustrous beauty, was wired with fear. Whether the troubled girl had affected the isolate cat, or the troubled cat had somehow affected the isolate girl we will never know. What we do know is that the two of them seemed fashioned of the same glistening grey, silvery cloth.

With the advent of Greyman, Lana began to stare, to look vacantly out at life, and to cease to be a participant as much as an avid observer. The use of drugs, however, lessened, to the point where I was pretty sure she wasn't using them anymore. In the weeks that followed, there was a marked improvement in Lana. Wherever she went one saw the shadow of blue-grey smoke at her feet. The girl and the cat were inseparable.

It happened, after her abstinence from drugs and a rather dramatic recovery, in which she just became more and more beautiful, that Lana fell in love with a certain young man. Now her attention to personal details became even more self-styled and intense. She began to carefully apply make-up and she dressed meticulously. Her natural beauty, always there, was now almost unbelievable. Lana and the cat, I think, had somehow managed to exchange selves.

Roger Caras in *A Celebration of Cats* tells a similar story about a caretaker cat who accomplishes a miraculous healing. This narrative involves a teenager, in some ways not unlike Lana, who has entered a world of dark shadows and overwhelming melancholy. His work went from worse to terrible at school, and his friends fell away one at a time. The boy was lonely, apparently frightened, and a pall of gloom seemed to have settled over him. He was being drawn down by an inexorable and as yet unidentified force.

The boy's condition worsened; he approached catatonia and, at fourteen, entered "a six-month-long tunnel of darkness and silence." The darkest period for the boy was when the youngster fell to a level where "the therapists ceased getting eye movement from him. He was frozen inside his own mind, and the specialists who came through had no explanation and held little hope."

There was one thing, however, that did offer a flicker of hope. The boy, Bobby, would move his eyes when shown the picture of a cat, and while there was no accompanying facial expression, the eyes were seen to move. Here, in Caras's words, is what transpired.

On a day well planned in advance, with his doctors and parents watching from behind a one-way window, a technician brought Bobby into a small examining room, seated him like the automaton he was in a straight wooden chair, then put a kitten in his lap. After a few moments Bobby tipped his head forward and looked down at the cat. Several minutes later he raised his hand in a voluntary action that had no parallel for months, hesitated, and then petted the cat. Some time later he tipped his head to one side, and this time there was a flicker of expression—not quite a smile, but something of recognition and reaction. His parents, standing behind the trick glass with Bobby's doctor, hugged each other and wept. After more than an hour alone with the cat, Bobby talked to it. His voice was flat, his speech monosyllabic—but this was an amazing giant step forward.

It was once believed that cats, having such acute sight themselves, could cure blindness in human beings. One way this was done was to place the paw of a live cat on the membrane of a blind person's eyes. The curative powers of the cat's pad were helpful in remedying sightlessness. Another cure was to use the eye fluid, or cat's tears, as they were called, for eyedrops.

Such premedieval medicines might or might not have worked, but the thought behind them remains with us today. We believe, more than ever, in the cat caretaker's mystical powers. Now, however, we call feline magic by other names: insight, intuition, empathy, and love. That is what brought Lazarus out of the darkness of his grave, and that is what makes the cat purr and pass on her well-being to us today.

The Lore of the Cat

The Russian Blue is one of the most elegant cats in the feline spectrum. Also known as the Archangel Blue, the Maltese, and the Spanish Blue, this lean, muscular cat with the long, articulate tail has fur like an extra layer of muscle with a mink's glistening sheen to it. The head is oval shaped with a well-developed muzzle. The cat has large, rounded ears and medium-sized oval eyes. The name, Archangel, seems to have come from the port of that name, where Russian sailors gathered up gray cats to sell in Great Britain during the 1800s.

Timid and reserved, the Russian Blue has a reputation for imprinting, or adapting, to one person. The intensity of the Blue's eyes is mesmerizing.

The gaze of the cat—healing, revealing, and sometimes annoying—was first observed and honored by the Egyptians. The earliest connection of cat psychic activity was also first recorded by them. They associated the cat with the hawk-headed god, Horus, who was the son of Isis. Legend has it that he could see around, and into, and above simultaneously.

We once had a Russian Blue who, after he grew quite old and was deaf, acted as if he always knew exactly what we were saying.

Moreover, this wily old tom could "see" visitors from afar—even before their arrival. A reclusive cat, he wanted no part of strangers and a full ten minutes before a car turned into our driveway, he would be seen slinking off to some corner where he'd be the observer and not the observed.

Dreaming, our Russian Blue wiggled his whiskers at advancing armies of mice. All cats do this, but our Blue sometimes rose from sleep, still adream, eyes half-lidded. Dreamers, these smoky beasts. Dreamers and seers and healers, each and every one.

The talismanic cat of the happy hearth visits virgins and blesses households. This comfy cat is very, very old—mythologically—dating back thousands of years.

Part of the myth is about the cat's preference for staying warm. Naturally, as cats warm themselves, they warm us, but not just on the outside.

The old Japanese cure for stomach cramps was a warm cat, but it was also used for both melancholy and epilepsy. In Scotland, it's still believed that cats can cure blindness. Cat skin and cat fur have been alternately used for burns, rheumatism, hives, and sore throats.

The most widely used cat item in healing has been the tail, for it is the bringer of balance—in Greek, *kattos* implies "tail waver," and thus has the cat wandered down the centuries, waving its tail at our illnesses, and, quite often, curing them.

THE CHESHIRE CAT

British Shorthair

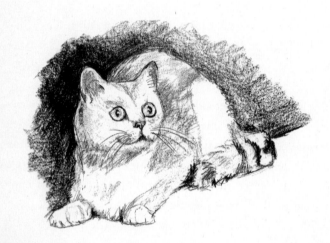

WHAT IS THERE about the image of the Cheshire Cat that affects our funny bone? Is it the disembodied smile, minus the cat's head, from which we get the expression "Cheshire Cat moon"? Is it the ringed tail, floating over Alice's head? Or perhaps it's the artful turn of phrase that the eccentric cat uses. Actually, it's all of these and more, but the most compelling feature is the Cheshire Cat's immanent grin: "The Cat only grinned when it saw Alice. It looked good-natured, she thought: still it had very long claws and a great many teeth, so she felt that it ought to be treated with respect."

Whether comic or mad, figment or fact, the Cheshire Cat is an interlude of classic invention, an exercise, some mathematicians claim, of much more than myth. Some say the fat cat in a tree is an expression of the new physics. Others remark that the cat is a philosophical separation, like a generation gap, set up in the late nineteenth century to haunt us today. If this is true, the cat and its argument with Alice is a metaphor for the collision between science and ethics. An argument, as we know too well, that is currently raging.

> "Would you please tell me, please, which way I ought to go from here?"
> "That depends a good deal upon where you want to get to," replied the Cat.
> "I don't much care where—" said Alice.
> "Then it doesn't matter which way you go," said the Cat.

The famous repartee of the lost girl and the found cat is full of references to math—the line, for instance. If you draw an unfinished line anywhere on a blank page it won't matter where the line goes, since it will always remain a line. Neither does it have a beginning or an ending. And when measured against absolute zero, or emptiness, the line that is a line expresses itself at zero, or infinity. If this sounds like double-talk, consider Alice's quandary. She wants to go "somewhere" and the Cheshire Cat tells her that surely she will, "if only you walk long enough." Just so, the journey of a line in space.

Alice's catty conversation with a celebrated English puss is one of the most commented-upon pieces of dialogue ever written. Its literary influence is pervasive. Even in Jack Kerouac's *On the Road* there's an echo of Alice's quandary:

> . . . we gotta go and never stop going til we get there.
> Where we going, man?
> I don't know but we gotta go.

Cheshire Cat myths include some pretty wacky metaphors, too. The Cat, some contemporary critics suggest, is the chaos of the universe. Others see the Cat as reason adrift in the world of unreason, or madness. ("We're all mad here. I'm mad. You're mad.")

The Cat, being born by Alice's dream in the beginning of the novel, is also a phantom presence of the unconscious. Carroll's controversial book has much to do with dreaming, and as readers, we can't help feel that we, too, are just another kind of dreamer ourselves. Lewis Carroll's personal diary, dated February 1856, sheds light on his interest in this question.

> When we are dreaming and, as often happens, have a dim consciousness of the fact and try to wake, do we not say and do things which in waking life would be insane? May we not then sometimes define insanity as the inability to determine which is the waking and which is the sleeping life?

The Cheshire Cat is a creature about whom we feel attraction and repulsion, friendliness and fear. We seem to like him and dislike him equally. We are not altogether sure how we feel about him. What the cat says *may* be true. On the other hand, it may not be true. Is this not the tenor of our time, envisioned by a visionary math teacher more than 130 years ago?

The Cat sets itself apart and asks a deceptively simple question, one that religion presses upon us and that science denies the validity of: "Where," the Cat asks, "are you going?" But the question isn't the thing that devils us; it's the belief that the Cat knows the answer and won't tell.

The Lore of the Cat

One cannot begin to tackle the breed of the Cheshire Cat without first checking the origin of its grin. The expression "to grin like a Cheshire Cat" probably came from the grinning cat faces on the signs of old country inns. But there is another theory that claims the famous English cheeses, fashioned to look like smiling cats, were the source of the grin and the phrase.

Think of it. The very idea of a cheese shaped like a cat . . . when the mouse got hold of it, he would, in effect, be devouring his arch-

enemy. This is the kind of situational pun that would have kept Carroll, an inveterate punster, in stitches.

Undoubtedly, the Cheshire puss most resembles a British shorthaired cat. In this case, it would be a heavily striped tabby—whether
orange and white, gray and white, black and gray is up to the imagination. John Tenniel, the famous Victorian illustrator, who provided
the pen and ink drawings, created a wide-faced, round-eyed cat with
a huge, thick tail and a great roundish body. The head is big with an
emphasis on the mouth, which is, of course, grinning. The nose is
short, broad, and stubby. The thick ears stand up prominently.

The Cheshire Cat, like all cats, is an allusion to the mythology
of Egypt, where the feline's eyes are a lunar symbol. The moon's
waxing and waning is visible in a cat's eye when subjected to light,
or the lack of it. And the cat itself, being accustomed to the night,
comes and goes as the moon rises and sets.

English critics have pointed out that the Cheshire Cat is like a
certain ghost cat. This one was at Congleton Abbey in Cheshire,
England, in the eighteenth century. It was often seen, sitting on a post
by the ruins of the abbey. When a person came upon it, the ghost cat
vanished into thin air. Was the Congleton Abbey spirit cat the inspiration for the Cheshire Cat? Some critics say that it was because Carroll's home was quite nearby Congleton. At the same time, many such
myths were rife in England at that time.

In Christian morality tales the cat is often a symbol for apathy
and forgetfulness. Thus, the Cheshire Cat's disconcerting and discon-
nected conversation with Alice; not once does the cat help her find
her way. Old European tales feature the forgetful cat and moralize
about it, saying that the only memory that is more fallible than a cat's
is that of a mouse. Since cats eat mice, this myth explains why cats
are elliptically minded—they dine upon forgetfulness!

Dale-Green author of *The Cult of the Cat*, explains that in Russia,
Jewish boys were once forbidden to touch a cat on the grounds that
they would lose their memory.

The Asian myth of the cat's knotted tail harks back to something
the cat forgot to do—to keep his mistress's rings from falling off his
tail; which is why all Siamese cats have a knotted tail to this day.

The Cheshire Cat is thought to be misanthropic—a cliché given to cats, in general. The so-called Gib cat of old England was an old tomcat, the veteran of fierce battles. Gib cats, though, were also neutered cats. Such a feline, it was said, found it difficult to laugh. If the Cheshire puss were one of these, his smile would be a false one, indeed, for he laughed at everything.

THE HOUSEHOLD CAT

All Breeds

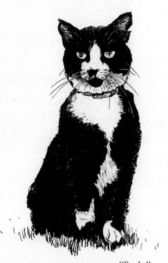

"Socks"

Most cats—if not all—have the ability to translocate, to find their home site after being irreversibly lost, by human standards. Researchers seek new information on the psychic cat, the so-called psi-trailing cat, but, really, all felines fall into this category when they are suddenly, or over a period of time, misplaced. And yet the subject remains pretty enigmatic—a sketchy, anecdotal thing at best. Indeed, how did Sugar, a black-and-white cat of mixed ancestry, travel from Anderson, California, to Gage, Oklahoma, a distance of 1,500 miles, on foot? The trip took fourteen months, but Sugar arrived home safely.

Frankly, no one knows, how Sugar did it, which broadens the mystery and expands the folklore of "homing" cats, whose travels admit to no obstacle whatsoever—neither weather, unfriendly terrain, nor physical stress, because, as the song goes, "The cat came back the very next day / the cat came back because he couldn't stay away."

Cats and dogs each have psi trailing, which stands for psychic tracking. Cats, however, seem to have the more finely honed talent of navigation. (Incidentally, the cat has an internal gyroscope in acrobatics, too: perhaps this is not an unrelated fact.)

Veterinarian Dr. Michael W. Fox has said that animals have a faculty that reduces "the dissonance between solar and internal time."

What this means, in terms of cats, is an affinity for the sun, an ability to "read" sunlight; to regard the time of day, the season of the year, the elapse of a second, through a subtle internal mechanism. So, possibly using solar and lunar magnetism, the cat may follow its translocational mind as unerringly as a map.

So, as the cat moves from one place to another, drawing ever closer to the place it wants to be, it reduces the stress that it feels, with regard to the area being traversed. In effect, the cat is saying to itself: "This way feels wrong, change direction; this way feels right, stay on target."

The cat, then, becomes a compact sonar finder, and it travels toward its destination swiftly, moving through inner, not outer, space.

The internal sonar theory, and the solar-dissonance theory, are but two possible explanations for psi trailing. There are of course a great many others, including this one from Joseph Wylder, author of *Psychic Pets*. His thought is that certain animals are capable of remarkable migrations on overcast days, and to do this they employ polarized light. Bees, for instance, distill light into a variant form that enables them to hone in on their hive without the aid of the sun. Light is thus converted into a kind of vibrational map.

Behaviorists suggest that cats, using their whiskers, set up an echolocation device. Indeed, they may even pick up magnetic impulses, perhaps from solar bodies, that affect their whiskers. Human beings have accomplished this with fillings in their teeth, so it doesn't seem illogical that a cat's whiskers act as receptors. (Not coincidentally, a "cat's whisker" is the receiver of a crystal radio.)

In occult cat lore, whiskers are things of great power. In vaudou, obeah, and Santeria, the cat's whisker is good for finding that which is lost. Cat's entrails were, and still are, used in some parts of the world for the purpose of prophecy; and cat's gut was once made into a string and used on such musical instruments as the ukulele. The "cat-gut leader," in fishing, was also quite common.

Joseph Wylder seems to think that the mystery of feline odyssey is not that different from animal migrations, in general. He believes that, in searching for what he calls a "quantitative bias" researchers often miss the point. What cannot be "measured, isolated, represented on a graph" is unreliable information. So how do we deal with the cat's cosmic compass?

Dr. Michael Fox, a scientist and a mystic, seems to have the best and most reasonable answer we've yet run across: "If an animal can perceive the time of day or the season, it should be able to find the square mile where it lives by 'reading' the sun and the angle of its rays in relation to the expected value that its internal clock anticipates. Incongruity is met with motivation to reduce the dissonance between solar and internal time. And the translocated animal is able to find his square mile on the globe."

Some would say even this is begging the issue; it still does not explain how blind, deaf, and severely impaired cats find their way against such odds as extreme weather and the obstacles of city walls and concrete impasses. So, the mystery shall probably always remain just that. Which is why the cat was once appointed to guide us into the next world.

The Lore of the Cat

Household pet may seem too broad a category, but it's necessary because, after reviewing the evidence of psi trailing, there's no particular breed that is an exception to the rule. Lost cats find their way home whether they are Persian, Russian Blue, or a mixture of Ragdoll and Egyptian Mau.

According to *The Reader's Digest Illustrated Book of Cats* the household pet, listed by them as if it were a special category, is

the alley cat, the farm cat, the cat from an animal shelter—
any cat without a pedigree or authenticated blood line.
Such cats are the basis for all the breeds that have come
about through careful breeding, mutations, and processes
of selection. Thanks to its native intelligence and adapta-
bility, the Household Pet has survived through the centuries—in spite of wars, diseases, and human cruelty.

The clairvoyant cat is Everycat. All cats remind us of the supernatural because of the moon's harvest cycle, and the feline sacrifices
that were made to ensure success in planting, growing, reaping. And
just as the Native American moon goddess was a fortune-telling
prophetess whose only friend was a cat, so, too, the pagan European
moon deity could tell the future and kept a cat for a pet.

According to Joseph Wylder, in *Psychic Pets,* the cat's connection
with the cosmos is somewhat determined by the moon, the supernatural, and "those parts of the universe which we humans fail to
understand." When the human race was closer to animals, in general,
we did obeisance to them, and, consequently, we shared their power.
No animal in the entire spectrum has been bowed to more times than
the cat; we honored her for the grace she gave us.

We cannot do honor to animals in zoos, petting gardens, or wild
habitats that are policed without losing much of our natural awe of
these creatures. Therefore, what some sociologists believe is that only
in our most easily monitored animals—cats and dogs—have we per-
mitted the pleasure of the "wild outside" to be part of our domesticated existence.

Our modern myths are full of surprises—cats, for instance who
are telepathic, and dogs who are psychic. We create a name, such as
psi trailing, for a phenomenon that, in our ancient history, was probably accepted behavior. The basic myth of the clairvoyant cat is that
its power surpasses our own. In appreciating feline traveler myths, we
accentuate our own potential as travelers. Once we, too, could travel
on a moonbeam merely by looking into a cat's eye. Though we
may content ourselves with tales of psi trailing, we permit ourselves

the luxury of imagining that we, too, could move through time and space without getting lost. Hopefully, the cat's confidence in us will continue to offer psychic guidance while unleashing our own powers. Then, and only then, will we return the cat's gift of intuitive grace.

THE BOBTAIL CAT

Manx

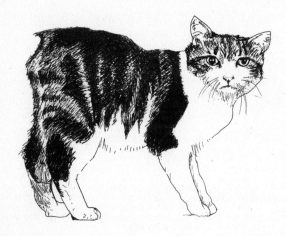

THE MYTHS OF the Manx go back to Noah's ark, and how the cat was late to board and, while apologizing for the delay, promised to pay for her keep. "I will catch mice to pay my way," the Manx told Noah. So he opened the hatch, she came slowly as cats are wont to do, and the hatch came down and cut off her tail. And thus did the bobtail come into being.

Another version of the same folktale is that the dog disliked the cat from the start and it was he who bit off her tail for spite. When the ark stopped at Ararat, the shamed cat ran off and, swam to the Calf of Man. The oft-quoted Noah myth goes like this:

> *Thus tailless Puss earned Mona's thanks*
> *And ever after was called a Manx.*

Tales from the Isle of Man, where the Manx is thought to have originated, have a distinctly Celtic flavor. For instance, cats who are put out at night and find their way in again are thought to have been let in by little people. But the myth doesn't stop there, for the king of the Manx is a housecat by day, and a little faery king by night. They say that he travels the lanes in a fiery carriage. Woe to the householder who has treated the cat king poorly that day, for when night comes, so, too, does the king's vengeance.

The American poet Ezra Pound had something to say about the lynx, if not the Manx, and used an Odyssean setting for his theme of the guardian cat.

> *O Lynx keep watch on my fire.*
> *Lynx, keep watch on this orchard*
> *O lynx keep the edge on my cider*
> *Keep it clear without cloud*
> *O lynx guard my vineyard*

Randall Jarrell also liked the lynx and one appears in *The Animal Family*. Here are a few of his observations that link the Manx with the northern bay lynx:

> The bigger he got, the stranger it was to see him in the rafters; set there in the air above their heads like a cloud by moonlight, staring at them with his big steady silver eyes, he looked magical, a spell the forest cast on the house.

Where is this mysterious island hopper, the Manx cat, actually from? Once again, the stories converge and diverge, leaving a cleaved tail, who knows where, but the commonly told legend is that two eighteenth-century ships were wrecked off the Isle of Man, by Spanish Point, near Point Erin. Reportedly, some desperate cats swam and climbed ashore.

However, a newspaper story that ran in 1801 said the following: "An East County ship was wrecked on Jurby Point, and a rumpy cat swam ashore." That leaves much to the imagination and little to pretense, but we don't get as much out of the incident as we do from the ark.

And, finally, there is this rendition from Reverend W. B. Clarke in *Cat Gossip Magazine*: "There was a Baltic ship in trouble, and as the vessel drew near to the shore, we saw a couple of tailless cats leap from the bowsprit, and these were the first of their kind ever to leave a pawprint on the sand of our Isle."

Geographically, the Manx cat has a pretty broad base and this breed, or something very much like it, has been seen in parts of Russia and even in the jungles of Burma. Malay Archipelago cats with "kinked, knotted, clubbed or otherwise malformed tails" are said by English scholar M. O. Howey to go back as far as 1783. The myth that accompanies their history suggests that a princess put gold rings on her cat's tail, but when the tail dropped, the rings went into the water. As a result, the princess knotted the cat's tail to prevent them from falling off again.

On the north coast of New Guinea, a native population that ate cats made it necessary for some cat owners to cut off their favorite pet's tail and bury it. That way, if the cat was stolen for food, the tail could be empowered to take the cat's owner to the cat itself.

Welsh stories of the Manx are rich in folkloric symbols. Robert Graves in the *The White Goddess* tells the myth of the great sow named Henwen, who was about to give birth. King Arthur, knowing that the magic pig was dangerous to Great Britain, drove Henwen into the sea, whereupon she blessed the nearby towns with her progeny.

These were grains of wheat, rye, and bees; a wolf pup and an eaglet; and, finally, a kitten. The cat was born in Arvon and was then thrown into the Menai Strait, where the sons of Palug fished it out and nursed it as their own. This became the celebrated Palug cat, the Manx.

The white sow, grain goddess of ancient Ireland and enemy of England, could change into a cat; and that, if any of the other myths are not satisfying, is why the Manx's tail is so short.

The Lore of the Cat

The Manx, which is a bobtailed domestic cat, has light fur, soft as a rabbit, with a dense undercoat. It wears a coat of many colors: solid, bicolor, tabby, marbled, tortoiseshell. Physically, the cat is muscular, short-backed, with the hind legs shorter than the front. The head is imposing, like that of a bobcat; the wide-set ears are slightly rounded. Confirmed mouser and outdoor hunter, the Manx is known as a playful, friendly cat, though it can be quite quirky as well.

The idea that this cat "differs from the ordinary cat little" may itself be a myth of sorts, since many owners believe the cat to be quite a lot different. Manx owner Janette Healy, who lives on an island, writes that her Manx is—not surprisingly—a boat cat.

> In the apartment complex that I operate with my husband, people check in for the weekend and dock their boats in our small harbour. Our Manx, Jack, enjoys watching the boats come in, and when a new one appears, he gives it his complete Coast Guard inspection. Jumping from the seawall or dock, he gets into the boat, going into the cabins and compartments. Then he jumps out and goes to the next newcomer, giving it his full attention. He never gets into the same boat twice, and some of our tenants have named him Captain Jack. The other Manx that we have is a 14 year old female named Zip, who for the first nine years of her life was strictly an indoor animal. Six years ago we changed the carpet in the house, and after that she wanted no part of the indoors ever again. Not even when there were thunderstorms, and believe it or not, hurricanes. You cannot upset a Manx's domain. Now she lives in the planter at the front of the house, and she's perfectly happy being an outside bush cat.

Since the Manx probably got its start on the Isle of Man by being brought aboard a Spanish galleon that was sunk off the coast, we imagine that other Spanish explorers brought along their tailless mousers, too. Ponce de Leon may have introduced an ancient strain of Manx to the barrier islands off the Gulf Coast of Florida. The pigs from his ships are still breeding on these islands 400 years later, and there are feral Manx cats on them as well. Who can say how long they have been there?

The Manx, regardless of its actual breed, reminds many people of the bobcat, and hence, the wildcat. The Hebrew word for wildcat is *haret,* from which we get the English Harry, a name, according to Dale-Green, that is associated with pillage and plunder. The old song "Just Wild About Harry" recalls this, as does the word itself, to harry someone, or something. Thus to "wildcat" a thing into submission.

THE DUPPY CAT

Jamaican Rampuss

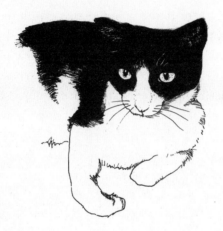

S PIRIT CATS HAVE been around since the domestication of wild felines in Libya and Nubia some 4,500 years ago. For, as we acquired the cat as a hunter and companion, we also acquired her for the art of sacrifice—to ensure that her beatific spirit would always be with us.

Ghost cats, then, are a spin-off from the belief that cat emissaries escorted human beings to the afterworld. The concept, a religion actually, was widely held from Egypt to Asia, and from the Mediterranean to the Caucasus. In the American South, there is a vast lore of spirit cat stories, most of which have grown out of African folk myths that go back to prebiblical Ethiopia.

One is about the Mississippi preacher who spends the night in a house that hasn't been occupied since the Civil War. He stays up all night reading the Bible. When he hears a noise, he looks down and sees a kitten by his foot. He tries to pat it, but his hand can't touch it, so he goes back to reading the Bible.

A little later, along comes another kitten, only this one's bigger than the first. Still, the preacher can't quite put his finger on it. When the next cat appears, it's larger still. After this, the cats keep getting larger and larger, until the great ghost cat of them all comes into the room.

Now the preacher lays down his Bible, goes to the window, and looks out; and he sees all the moony ghost cats in the whole world pouring into that haunted house. They are hissing and spitting and spatting and growling. Soon, someone comes to that house, discovers the preacher there, lying flat out on the floor, unconscious.

The rescuer brings the preacher home and puts him in his bed, and the preacher wakes up with a start and sings:

> *"Oh, Lord, I feel like a feather in the air,*
> *I feel like I never prayed a prayer.*
> *Oh, Lord, the cat's in the cupboard, the cat's in the sink*
> *the cat's got my tongue, and I can't even think."*

"The Preacher and the Cat" is a well-known southern folktale. Notice that the cats are not featured as enemies or adversaries in this instance—they are simply ghosts. Much of our ghost-cat mythology runs along the same course—cats that intimate the end, cats who are pass-over spirits, cats who appear when we are ready to walk the passageway between life and death. The preacher, in this case, got a liberal does of his own spiritual medicine, an extra dose of "nightshade du *chat*."

Once, in Jamaica, we were staying in the old quarters of an estate, a place well frequented, we were told, by duppies, or ghosts. One night we had a feline visitor, a scarred and scratched up old tomcat, whom everyone called Rampuss.

This cat had never been domesticated, but every now and then, it briefly took up residence with someone. The first night we saw Rampuss, we fed him, and after that, he stayed with us for a week.

During that time, everyone said that there were duppies just falling out of the trees. The cook said it was the fault of the cat, because cats like duppies and duppies like cats, and that's the way it's been since the beginning.

M. O. Howey devotes a chapter to spirit cats in *The Cat in Magic*. One of her tales concerns English Egyptologist Lord Carnarvon at Thebes a century ago. Having found a cat's coffin in a tomb, Lord Carnarvon took it home with him and placed it in his bedroom so that he could look at it in the morning.

> A branch of a tree was swaying in the night breeze outside,
> and its shadows danced to and fro over the face of the cat,
> causing the yellow eyes to open and shut, as it were, and
> the mouth to grin.

Under the glittery gaze of this three-thousand-year-old mummified cat, Lord Carnarvon went to sleep, but he was awakened by a pistol shot. When he got up to find what the commotion was about, he discovered the mummy case had cracked open to reveal the cat with the swathing cloth unraveling about its neck.

Suddenly, a ghost cat jumped into the air, landed on the bed, and raked Carnarvon's hand with its claws.

Carnarvon ran to the window where he saw his "own pet tabby, standing with arched back and bristling fur, glaring into the bushes as if she saw ten feline devils therein."

Carnarvon said that "the events I have related can be explained in a perfectly natural manner if one be inclined to do so." Let those inclined, be so inclined; as for us, we would rather imagine the event than think about it, or try to explain it.

The connection, though, between cats and the afterworld is so deeply engraved in the human imagination that cats are expected to envision things that we only dream about. For instance, the other day a cat lover, Joanne Merritt, sent us this story.

> Years ago our daughter, Mary, died. One of the last things
> she did before passing on was to make Christmas orna-

ments for our tree. And every year, in her honor, when Christmas comes we remember her by decorating the tree with her little baubles. This year, for some reason, we found that our cat, Peppy, would not leave these orna-ments alone. He would remove them from the tree and hide them. We went from room to room, looking for those lost ornaments of Mary's. When I placed them back on the tree, Peppy would go about his routine, usually at night, of removing and hiding. As Christmas drew near, however, he left these hand-made decorations alone and was satisfied to lie down under the lights and smile up at us the way cats do.

The spirit cat is not just a cat spirit, but it truly reflects the spiritual nature of the animal. For the cat is poised between two worlds: night and day, mind and matter, body and soul. And what the cat does for humanity, and has always done, is to let us know that the two worlds are really one.

The Lore of the Cat

Rampuss is the Jamaican name for any good-size stray male cat who likes to have things go his own way. All rampuss variants are probably descended from the British shorthaired cat, but they have a particularly Jamaican quality, owing to the fact they've lived in that country since the seventeenth century.

Jamaicans do not really trust cats, as evidenced by the expression "You can't tell the puss until you put out the butter." However, the African identification with the largest of cats, the lion, is omnipresent in the Caribbean, and in Jamaican Rastafarian circles, the lion is the spiritual center, the soul, of a man. In *The African-American Alphabet* by Gerald Hausman and Kelvin Rodriques, the power of the lion comes from pulpits that rang with the clamor of lionization in parable, song, and sermon. Daniel in the lions' den; David's body-guard, who slew a lion; the lion-faced warriors of God; the princely tribe of Judah proclaiming a lineage of lions. We still speak metaphorically of bearding the lion and it is in the face of the Pharaoh that we may also see the lion's almond-eyed likeness and the false beard upon the shaven chin. Part falcon, part cobra, part lion, he was brother-god to those who lent him their skin and eye and facile brain. As a noble figure, he was irresistible; on the battlefield he was immortal. Moreover, as African-Americans under-stand today, the Pharaoh was black.

The lion, then, is a masculine figure, forged by symbiosis with the sun. The man, or woman, who assumes this religious stance, as in Rastafarianism, borrows the lionlike heraldry of Haile Selassie I, King of Kings, Lord of Lords, Conquering Lion of the tribe of Judah.

This occultism of the lion reminds us of a time when the cat, like the Sphinx fashioned after her, could see beyond life and death, past and present, to that bright dream of the future.

The Immortal Cat

Abyssinian

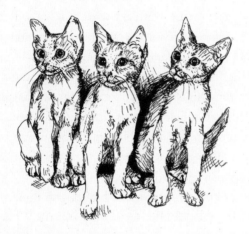

P ERHAPS THE OLDEST of feline archetypes is that of the immortal cat, the goddess, who sits beside the demons of disaster and wisely, patiently guides the anxious human soul to its destiny. Unlike the caretaker cat, the martyr cat, the healing cat, and the spirit cat, this archetype is really the nurse of the next experience. The immortal cat exists, then, in the netherworld between life and death, watching and waiting, passive until the moment when the human spirit is to be set free. Then, and only then, will she lead the human soul to its final place of rest. This is the myth of the immortal cat.

One of the finest examples of the myth comes from the pen of Tennessee Williams. The story is called "The Malediction" and it is about an unlucky man named Lucio and a female cat, whose name is Nitchevo. The fate that closes in on the lonely stranger, the misplaced, panicky little Lucio, who is a metaphor for modern man, is one of inevitable disaster.

Williams casts the landscape, the buildings, the desperate people of the town, in a compact of human suffering. This, we are told, is the Middle Ages, that dark time when cats were executed for being agents of evil. Actually, the drama is set in the mid-fifties of industrial America, which has a medievalism all its own.

As Lucio looks out at the world, the world looks in on him, darkly, cruelly. We are given the impression of the coming collision, the apocalypse, but we are not told what it is, or why it is coming, only that it will bring more sorrow. As the old cat goddess is invoked, we see the end of the millennium as the poet W. B. Yeats in "The Second Coming" saw it: the great cat beast slouching toward Bethlehem, the whirling birds circling above it, the world spinning out of control, the ultimate epoch of chaos close at hand. Williams describes the end of the earth, as if it had all happened before, and as if it would happen again, and he gives it particular meaning through the eyes of the little "Everyman" named Lucio.

Lucio is a figure of doom, but he has one thing on his side— his faithful, immortal cat, Nitchevo. This animal, Williams explains, is the first thing in that despairing town to have an "asking look" and to possess a modicum of innocence. In time, the cordiality of the cat warms the little man's heart and a love grows between them which, the reader supposes, is not something that will be easily, if ever, broken apart. And that is because it is a myth, one that came from Egypt 4,500 years ago, one that is not perishable.

It is the ominous title "The Malediction," that reminds us of doom and defeat. Will the cat turn out, after all, to be an emissary of darkness? No, because Nitchevo is a symbol of the great cat mother, whose mythos is watchfulness over the anxious human soul. The cat's watchfulness rivals that of the sun and the moon because, in effect, it is each of these itself. In the tale, though, the cat strays; and the straying cat and the fraying man share the same fate, death. They, we understand, are not mismatched but misplaced—born in the wrong century, born out of time.

Nitchevo, alone, knows what human fate and feline fate have in

store for them. The medium through which human birth is blessed
and death is transfigured is something that Nitchevo understands. It
is the goddess in her. Still, a dire fate awaits each, and they cling to
one other until Lucio gets lost and Nitchevo strays, searching for him.

In the last few lines of the story, Nitchevo and Lucio are reunited, as Fate had wanted them to be, and they are bonded in a crucial,
sacrificial act. Here we see that the drowning cat is part of a purifi-
cation rite, a passage to the next world.

> He knew she could not go on living. She knew it, too.
> Her eyes were tired and dark; eclipsed in them now was
> that small, sturdy flame which means a desire to go on and
> which is the secret of life's heroic struggle. No, the eyes
> were eclipsed.

One knows that this eclipse is the Middle Ages, the desecration
of the cat as goddess. Time is compressed in this myth, all time seem-
ing to exist at once. So Nitchevo, who lives in the past as a goddess,
and as a witch's familiar, knows full well what is happening—the
burnings, the beheadings, the betrayal of she who was humanity's
savior.

All of this Nitchevo knows. She is timeless; she is Christ on the
cross asking the Father, "Why hath thou forsaken me?" And she is
the numinous mystery on the banks of the Nile, casting a shadow as
large as the river is long; she is the slouching beast, the Antichrist,
coming at the culmination of Revelation.

As the sun sinks in a skein of flame, Lucio and Nitchevo perish
together in the dirty, oily river beside the muted, desecrated town.
She struggles against him, but only briefly. She knows what she must
do. Then, as they sink beneath the town, the smoke, the wind, and
the water, Nitchevo feels their communal immersion, man and cat,
become a benediction.

Lucio's last words prefigure not death but some unknowable,
transfigural realm, some glimpse of rebirth: "Soon, soon, very soon."
The words close, like water lapping, like a cat licking, like the tapping
of an egg about to break open.

The Lore of the Cat

The Egyptian Mau, a breed that naturally occurs in Egypt, was carved in ivory and lapis and cast in bronze in 1400 B.C.E. Here is the goddess cat with a gold ring in her nose, with another on one ear, and with an owl pendant gleaming on her breast. Modern Maus have been bred to resemble this ancient prototype—a cat with sapphire eyes, a flexible body made of sinew and silk.

The Mau is first cousin of the Abyssinian. A temple cat whose image was immortalized in carnelian and agate, the Mau was caught by Egyptian artisans in every conceivable mood—crouching, prowling, walking, pouncing. They portrayed her in full flight, chasing sparrows, and deep asleep, yet wakefully dreaming.

The dominant marking pattern is spots, separate and seemingly random. The face is narrow, doglike, triangular, with mascaraed outlining around the eyes. She comes in three colors—silver, bronze, and smoke—and the fur is fine and silky, and not dense enough to keep the cat warm in colder climates. The tail is long and tapered and the overall posture of the Mau is supremely statuesque.

Cats have suffered two primary sacrificial fates: fire and water. Hundreds of thousands of cats were burned, drowned, and beheaded in Europe and America during the times of feline genocide (from the plague years through the Puritan period). In Germany, France, and England, cats were burned for sacrificial reasons, and their ashes were scattered in the cornfields to ensure the fecundity of the crop. Part of the symbolism of the watchful cat that never dies is this: the cat is wedded to the earth by sacrifice. In primitive terms, sacrifice means "to give up" and it is not to be confused with ritual murder.

Medicinally, cat burnings were sometimes enacted to create the smoke of "second sight." For instance, the Talmud tells how to burn the placenta of a mother black cat, turn it into powder, and rub this well into the eyes. The cat's association with fire, historically, is Egyptian, and patterned after sun worship. Yet, throughout postplague Europe, the hearth cat was thought to be a thing of beauty beyond homeyness. As cats ensured crops, they also ensured homes.

Fire cats go back into our prehistory, but what of water cats? They, too, harken back to sacrificial libations. Water as the element of rebirth (as in the ritual of Christian baptism) and the cat as a symbol of immortality go well together. In one of our oldest myths, the water of the great Flood cannot touch the cat, who jumps ship, the ark, and still lives to tell about it.

During the ceremonies in honor of Bastet, the Egyptian women raised their dresses over their heads and sang out loud bawdy tales to the accompaniment of the crotala, archaic cymbals. All along the Nile, the procession of barges carried men and women to their appointed place at Bubastis, where the statue of Bastet was brought forth and given her due in prayer, song, and ceremony. This was known, incidentally, as "the Coming Forth" and it was a rite that permanently infused a sense of sexual power into the cat.

Some 1,300 years later, the cat's emergence as a water figure capable of invoking the powers of nature occurs in Germanic and Celtic legends, as the sea cat, an octopuslike deity whose dark force controls the underworld of the sea in opposition to Neptune. This is Ursula, the Sea Witch in the popular animated Disney feature *The Little Mermaid*. She is the sexual water cat, who enslaves lovers and consigns human souls to the underworld.

It is amazing to think that this myth has survived intact after so many thousands of years, for it's little more than Ra, the cat, and Apep, the snake, battling for the dominion of day and night.

THE TRAVELING CAT

Siamese

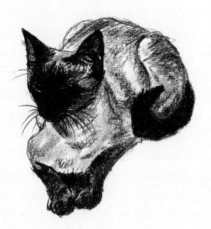

SOME CATS ARE naturally good traveling companions, while others suffer apoplexy at the mere sight of a suitcase. Cleveland Amory, author of *The Cat Who Came for Christmas,* speaks of his white cat, Polar Bear, going with the author to Hollywood, and how his friends warned him against "feline foraying." The reason given was that "cats ranked as a fellow traveler on long trips somewhere above alligators and orangutans."

Amory comments that cats are territorial, and that his cat "didn't like anything happening that didn't happen before"—something that, most of us would agree, is a feline tendency. As Amory reminds us, too, the simple luxury of a hotel room is often missed by the feline visitor, for whom the room is an "uncharted wilderness, around any corner of which lurked dangers which would put to shame a Chamber of Horrors in a wax museum on Hallowe'en."

Of course, what's good for the cat isn't always good for the puss; which to to say that all cats are not the same. Some experts, and Cleveland Amory is one, believe that most cats can accept dislocation, provided it was part of their early training. There must be—to the cat's unwavering eye—a method to our madness; for cats and dogs alike are very big on procedure.

Here, then, are some cases in point that seem to defy the norm of the feline traveler's bias. These are cats who don't mind a bump in the road, who, in fact, don't mind the road. Some actually crave it. A black-striped gray cat we heard about was carried around in a large basket wherever he went from the age of three months.

The cat's name was Samuel Tinker, and as long as he was in his basket, he was in high clover. He stretched out in it, too, full length, and whether or not he was skipping across the bounding main on a luxury liner, hanging out in a down-at-heels hotel, or passing through the clamorous cobblestoned streets of a Turkish bazaar, he was perfectly at ease. Samuel was an exemplary feline forayer, and at the height of his career as a traveling cat, he even learned to swim behind a gunboat in a seaport off the North China Coast.

Another remarkable road bum was a fifteen-pound Siamese whom writer Michael Joseph took with him to Burma. The cat, whose name was Billikin, traveled on trains, survived fires, and at one point escaped from the clutches of a Burmese panther. To the cat's credit, she did it all with a smile.

Perhaps the most amazing of Joseph's traveling felines was the Persian whose rounds about Persia were made on the back of a donkey. The cat accepted this form of travel so readily that when camp broke, and the donkeys were being packed, she'd await the appropriate moment, then fly to the packsaddle in anticipation of her journey. All day she rode along the trail, as content as, well, a cat.

Normally, cats do not mind movement if they can "see with their nose." Such is not the case with an animal shut up in a box where unfamiliar smells lead to the chamber of horrors of a cat's fertile imagination.

Ernest Thompson Seton, author of *Wild Animals I Have Known,* once stated that a cat carefully examines "the long, invisible, coloured stream the wind is made of." Our cat, Sammie, who, though all black, was a three-quarter Siamese, would check the stream of wind one bright morning and, finding it to her liking, light out upon the road for three to four months—always to return, however, with a seasonal change, or a shift in the weather.

One day a friend of ours, who lived miles away from us, phoned to say, "I think your cat is over at our barn." We drove over there, and there was Sammie, our Siamese. She wasn't a bit glad to see us. We took her with us, and while she said nothing in the car, she looked displeased. When we deposited her in the kitchen of our home, Sammie headed for the back door, which was slightly ajar, and sniffing the wind but once, she was on the road again.

When Sammie did return, sometimes after as many as six months, she would sing (purr) for days on end. All she did was walk around the house, singing, "I'm back, isn't it wonderful? I'm home."

By nightfall, the singing became more modulated, but it still went on for at least a couple of days. Of course, one bright morn when the sky turned a certain indefinable hue and there was some kind of minty freshness on the wind, Sammie would bestir herself, sniff that invisible stream of destiny, and disappear for perhaps another six months. One morning, after fifteen years of parting and returning, Sammie left, never to come back.

Fortunately, we had Moonie, Sammie's seal point son. Moonie never left the house except under extreme duress. He was exactly like Amory's Polar Bear, a nontraveler, or a traveler in the mystic realms of the mind. When it was necessary to move Moonie from the mountains of New Mexico to the pinewood flats of Florida, this feline studied the move from one remove, his face firmly resolved not to budge.

As each article of familiar furniture was lifted from its characteristic place, Moonie let out a Siamese yowl. Finally, when everything went off in a moving van, Moonie settled down into a disconsolate mood. We had a cat-traveler's box for him, one of those claustrophobic little prisons, and after a brief struggle, Moonie settled in and accepted his fate.

In each new hotel room, Moonie was allowed to leave his jail-house, and he could move about at will, but he didn't; he stayed put, usually hopping onto our bed and immediately crawling under the covers, where he stayed for the duration of the night.

Actually, our blue-fronted Amazon parrot, George, saw more of the passing countryside than Moonie, and he talked about it more, too. Moonie never said a blessed, or unblessed, word until, after a thousand miles, we got to southwest Florida. Then he yowled quite a bit, presumably telling us of the horror he'd been through at our behest.

Moonie did not like the subtropical atmosphere he'd been forced to live in. Normally an ebullient cat, he grew very glum. He didn't like it. He wanted his old home back; we could see it on his face. He wanted the familiar smells; he hated Florida.

Within a few weeks of arriving in the Sunshine State, Moonie came down with a bad cold, a cough that lingered through the winter. Then one morning we noticed that he had visibly changed. His lovely dark chocolate mask had a frostiness in it. Moonie was going white in the face. In one night this cat had aged ten years. He blinked dimly when we spoke to him, and we could hear him saying, "Go away."

Then we got an idea fostered by Ernest Thompson Seton's remark about the invisible stream of wind a cat is dependent upon, and we took Moonie outside for walks with us. We showed him the bright green world of palms and palmettos and we let him sniff the invisible stream that had guided his mother for so many years.

Vaguely, after several outdoor experiences, Moonie began to grow more cheerful. His eyes grew brighter. Each morning he went outside and drank the wind. It was spring and there were orange blossoms on the air. We took Moonie to the dock beside our house, and a soft-shelled turtle arose from the dark, tea-colored water. Moonie met the turtle; they practically touched noses.

In no time at all, Moonie settled back into his old ways, comfortable, at last, with this major move from one place to another. He became his old talkative self. He grew strong and confident, and although he was sixteen years old, and looking a bit paunchy, he trimmed down and started to look fit. Most amazing, his mask lost the frost; it got dark again, the color of German chocolate.

Today when people see Moonie, they imagine he is two or three years old. No one guesses his real age. Sometimes we wonder why human beings cannot do what Moonie did—turn back the years and grow young again. When things get us down, when life seems to be out of control, as it was for our Siamese cat, why can't we just take a deep draft of wind, and follow that invisible stream toward our destiny?

The Lore of the Cat

The Siamese was, at one time, a wild species in the Far East, but we have no proof of this. The first Siamese in literature occurs in a five-hundred-year-old manuscript in the National Library at Bangkok, Thailand. King Chulalongkorn (the son of Monkut, whose story is told in *The King and I*) presented a pair of seal point Siamese cats named Pho and Mia to the British consul in Bangkok. This began the Western era of the breed, early in the nineteenth century.

Dark of face and blue-eyed, this chocolate-and-cream-colored cat is as distinct in form as in reputation. Walt Disney's characterization in the cartoon *Lady and the Tramp* presents two Siamese cats of cold, conniving, contrary personality. Nothing, however, could be further from the truth, in terms of breed, for these empathic felines are beautiful to look at and to be around and they are anything but mean-spirited.

The Siamese is a finely boned and well-muscled cat, with a tail which is long and thin. The proud, wedge-shaped head bears regally the ancient lineage of this highborn animal. The ears are quite large, and yet proportionate, and the eyes are almond shaped, and the fur short and fine.

There are four kinds of Siamese: the seal point, the blue point, the chocolate point, and the lilac point. These designations refer to the relative darkness of the extremities—face, ears, tail, and feet.

Siamese cat myths often tell of humans whose souls have stayed for a time in the body of this royal cat. It is a cat of longevity, and a cat that confers longevity to its owner. Siamese cats don't like to be patronized or trifled with, and their wish is to be with one person, or perhaps two people, at a time. Once, in its long history, the Siamese cat was the guardian of the king of Siam's children, and this accounts for the diversity in the cat's vocalization. No cat has more to say than does the Siamese. If you do not talk to this cat, he will challenge you to do so. Our Siamese will actually put his paw to our lips to make us talk when he thinks we're being too quiet. He simply demands that we speak to him.

Our cat speaks in rounded vowels. Alone, annoyed or dissatisfied, he may let out some strange yowls, but this is true to form; all members of the breed do this as a way of letting out feelings about food, family, friends, anything that is weighing on the mind.

Cats may be the original aromatherapists of the animal world. Aromatherapy is an ancient healing art which came from Asia, the continent of the Siamese cat. The spirit of place, from which we humans achieve a sense of deep rest, can be nurtured through smells. Certain scents bring us back to who we are and meditatively return us to well-being.

If we, whose sense of smell is considerably less than the cat's, can find harmony in the moment of a particular fragrance, then the feline's appreciation must be a thousand times greater. A cat needs to "know" with its nose as much as, if not more than, a dog. For the cat, the nose evaluates more than smell; it takes in mood, time, climate, energy, mind; every nuance that possibly exists on the plane of the present moment can be experienced by a cat's ultrasensitive nose, palate, facial receptors, and whiskers. When a cat is in the "know," and all of these factors are working smoothly, the cat is content. However, when in rapid transit, as our Siamese Moonie was, the knowing is reduced—in a moment—to forgetting.

THE LITERARY CAT

British Shorthair

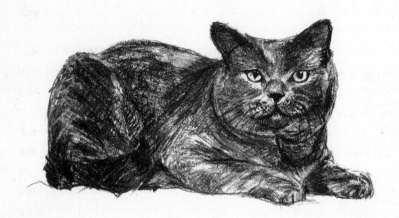

THE FIRST LITERARY genre to feature the cat was the animal fable, the most famous of which was written by Aesop in the sixth century B.C.E. The bestiary followed sometime in the fourth century. It was really the first natural history ever written, appearing first in Greek and later in Latin. La Fontaine, the seventeenth-century French fabulist, was intrigued by cats, placing their intelligence above dogs and uncomfortably close to humans.

From that time on, writers have had a field day with the literary cat. Countless poets, playwrights, and fantasists have polished their pens on the contradictory nature of *Felis*. Today, the writer's cat is as much a breed as the literary cat is a soft-footed, feline genre. Both may be a bit overworked sometimes, but writers do turn out great books about great cats.

Ernest Hemingway wrote about his cats frequently, and in Cuba, his farm cats rose into the high teens in number. In her book, *The Florida Keys,* Joy Williams writes;

It was at the Finca (nine miles outside of Havana) where the ghastly collection of inbred cats roamed and not in Key West, where the pet population, which numbered several peacocks, included only two cats, one of which the children once dyed a dark green, producing unknown consequences.

Today, however, the Hemingway House Museum in Key West has fifty resident polydactyl cats. These are of the extra-toed variety, but no one locally calls them polydactyl: they're simply called conch cats. Supposedly, sailors in the New World considered six-toed cats to be good luck charms. Hemingway was given one of these back in the thirties by a ship captain, and some of the museum cats, according to the museum directors, are descendants of that original feline.

Hemingway loved cats, all kinds. He called them "cotsies" and in one of his letters to Charles Scribner Sr. he said, "Dogs are trumps but cats are longest suit we hold." In his fiction, he often used that long suit to his advantage.

Boise, the cat who was Hemingway's best friend in Cuba, appears in his novel *Islands in the Stream.*

This big, rangy black tomcat cared for no others of his kind, barely tolerating his own son, Goats. And the only thing that he doesn't do with Hudson (Hemingway's alter ego in the novel) is drink with him.

Eat with him, he does indeed: "he ate everything the man ate especially all of those things cats would not touch." This included chilled mango slices as Boise and Hudson breakfasted together. And, for dinner, halves of *aguacate,* or alligator pear, filled with dressing of oil and vinegar.

One night Boise observes Hudson walking with Boise's son, Goats. Boise does not approve, looking on coolly as Hudson and Goats walk under the dark green leaves.

Hemingway writes that Goats is "a big-shouldered, heavy-necked, wide-faced, tremendous-whiskered, black, fighting cat" who seems to have a special feel for human language.

Medicine was a magic word with Goats and as soon as he heard it, he lay on his side to be stroked. "Remember the medicine? the man asked him and the big cat writhed in his hardy rough delight."

The story is that early one morning when Hudson is suffering from a hangover of the deadly double-frozen daiquiris served at the Floridita in Havana, Goats helps him find the big double Seconal capsule under the bed, and from that time on, the cat with the unbeaten head of a lion shares a moment unblessed by the presence of the chosen one, Boise. This medicine-retrieval business is his own, and not to be taken lightly. For whenever Hudson even mentions the word, Goats purrs loudly in sweet remembrance: "Goats loved the sound of the word, which symbolized all this rich life he was sharing, and purred stronger than ever."

However, although the medicine ritual is purely Goats's dominion, all else falls to the black-masked Boise. Of his cat, Hemingway once said in an interview with Lillian Ross,

"I have a cat named Boise, who wants to be a human being," he went on slowly, lowering his voice to a kind of grumble. "So Boise eats everything human beings eat. He chews vitamin B Complex capsules, which are as bitter as aloes. He thinks I am holding out on him because I won't give him blood-pressure tablets, and because I let him go to sleep without Seconal." He gave a short, rumbling laugh. "I am a strange old man," he said. "How do you like it now, gentlemen?"

Ernest Hemingway is best known as a writer's writer, who had the power to walk into a room and draw all of the oxygen out of it. His persona was often violent, frequently peevish, and always competitive. The softer side of Hemingway, say the people who knew him, came out when he was with his cats.

One time on the Central Highway he had seen a cat that had been hit by a car and the cat, fresh hit and dead, looked exactly like Boy. His back was black and his throat, chest, and forefeet were white and there was the black mask across his face. He knew it couldn't be Boy because it was at least six miles from the farm; but it had made him feel sick inside and he had stopped the car and gone back and lifted the cat and made sure it was not Boy and then laid him by the side of the road so nothing else could run over him. The cat was in good condition, so he knew he was someone's cat, and he left him by the road so they would find him and know about him rather than have to worry about him. Otherwise he would have taken the cat into the car and had him buried at the farm.

Hemingway was just one of many twentieth-century writers who spent a lifetime among cats. Colette, the French novelist, wrote a novel about her cat, and posed as a feline on the cover herself. In fact, many women writers have touched the cat's whisker to fiction, but actually, more men have crossed over the old cat cemeteries of the past in their writing, and Hemingway was no exception to this rule. He could be catty or catatonic, by turns, but he always strove for catlike perfection in his writing.

The Lore of the Cat

From the description given, Boise is a British, or American, shorthair. The head is broad with well-developed cheeks and a relatively short nose. The ears are of medium size, rounded at the tips, and the eyes are medium to large, and set well apart. This is a cat we have all seen and some of us have owned, and he can be quite large (as in the case of Goats), but usually he is smaller in stature (as in the case of Boise).

The colors of the cat range from black and tabby to bicolors. The fur is plush, dense, and generally longer than other members of the shorthair family.

The British shorthair is so self-sufficient that it sometimes seems utterly aloof. An excellent hunter, the cat may behave in a manner befitting one—staying outdoors and constantly on the prowl. An outdoor cat, the British shorthair has an allegiance like that of a good hunting dog to one primary owner.

There are a lot of reasons why the cat figures heavily in our literature. Saki, Kipling, Baudelaire, Poe—so often male writers have gone in for the feline attribute. Clearly, there are answers in the fact that writers, male in particular, need the benign anima of the cat to figure things out. Puss in Boots frees his forlorn master from spiritual bondage by teaching him to see with a cat's cunning eye. Psychologists have commented that men often find cats alluring because they possess the inner wisdom, the insight of women, but that men are also afraid of cats for this same reason.

Perhaps it is not too much of an exaggeration to say that men need cats the same way that cats need mice—it's a survival thing, and it goes back a long while. When the end comes, if it ever does, most assuredly the cat, plus a few of her friends, will be there. Whatever human beings think of their ability to survive, the cat does it better, and has done it longer. Carl Van Vechten explains that, after the apocalypse, there will still be the cat.

> He will bridge the gap until man appears again, and then he will sit on new hearths and again will teach his mighty lesson to ears and eyes that again are dumb and blind. Shylock's doom was foretold by Shakespeare from the moment the poet asked the poor creature to say, "The harmless necessary cat." For it is possible, nay probable, that the cat, unlike man who forgets his previous forms, remembers, really remembers many generations back; that what we call instinct may be more profound than knowledge.

THE COON CAT

Maine Coon

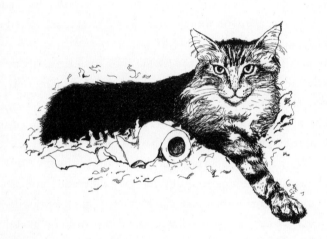

OF ALL CREATURES who came from the wild and who have supposedly been tamed no single animal has been more resistant than the cat. True or false?

If true, the cat within our walls is still an outsider; if false, the poor maligned kitty deserves an apology. The point is that some wild part of us, of human beings, seems to require a permanent part of the wilderness in the house, the apartment, the room where we live.

And the cat, ruffled and reckless when it comes to being pushed around, is not above reminding us of our own rough-edged origins. How does this anthropology fit into the mythology of cats? More than likely, it explains our fascination with, our passion for cat breeds, especially those that resemble the leopard, as in the spotted ocicat, or the Maine coon cat, which legend tells is part raccoon and part wild-cat.

What we truly know of the coon cat is that it is the first long-haired breed to have emerged naturally in North America.

This large cat came from nonpedigree Persian stock and his origins can be traced as far back as the 1700s. Ship captains, traveling from Ankara, Turkey, to the seaports of New England brought the Maine coon's ancestor as a curiosity and a pet for their wives. Legend has it that some of these cats took to the pine woods, especially in Maine, and particularly on some of the islands, and thence mated there with wild raccoons.

Maine natives claim that the Maine coon's wildness, ringtail, and size prove the myth is accurate. But, although it has merit as myth, it is not the least bit scientific as fact.

The Maine coon did, however, get loose in the islanded upper reaches of the Penobscot Bay, and there is ample proof that a "pure strain" of Maine coon occurred there sometime in the last fifty years.

These cats have appeared in over sixty different color patterns, they are usually large—the males can be up to eighteen pounds—and they have a dense outer coat suitable to a damp winter climate.

Although the standard Maine coon is thought to be amiable and affectionate, the old legend of the islands maintains that this cat is ardently individualistic and rather antisocial. An example of this myth is found in John Steinbeck's *Travels with Charley*.

> For George is an old gray cat who has accumulated a hatred of people and things so intense that even hidden upstairs he communicates his prayer that you will go away. If the bomb should fall and wipe out every living thing except Miss Brace, George would be happy. That's the way he would design a world if it were up to him. . . . I am told that when guests sleep in the house George goes into the pine woods and watches from afar, grumbling his dissatisfaction and pouring out his dislike. Miss Brace admits that for the purposes of a cat, whatever they are, George is

worthless. He isn't good company, he is not sympathetic, and he has little esthetic value.

On the basis of this short paragraph, we actually drove from New Jersey to Deer Isle, Maine, where Steinbeck had met George, in search of, not a real cat, but a palpable myth. We found it, too. The cats were there all right, carefully hoarded by islanders. No outsider could buy one, not in 1963. They were not, as Steinbeck professes later in his narrative, of the Manx tailless variety; rather they had full, fluffy tails.

The Maine coons we saw on Deer Isle were almost bobcat size, and they could vault five feet in an impressive vertical leap, and furthermore, the pure strain, according to the islander we stayed with, traditionally had seven toes. None of this legendary equipage is mentioned in any of the breed books—nor are the taillessness, the misanthropy, the wild, untamable qualities put forth by Steinbeck. In truth, it's all part of a wonderful myth, and not surprising when you consider that John Steinbeck was one of the nation's greatest mythmakers.

The coon cat, as we found out, was a perfect candidate for mythologizing. With tufted ears and widely set apart eyes, the cat who lived with us was nothing if not fantastical. This one's name was Mitzi and she had a raccoon's curiosity, a lynx's ferocity. She did have the seven toes and with her snowshoe-shaped feet, her footfalls were anything but quiet.

In addition, there were other little flashes of the wilderness in Mitzi's demeanor. She liked to hold food in her paws—quite raccoonlike, actually—and she was unafraid of water.

During the winter months, she walked on crusted snow, and a night never passed when this cat did not go outside to hunt in the prickly balsam woods that edged the property.

Altogether this is a multifaceted cat, an exceptional beauty, who has a host of myths surrounding her mystique.

On the day we were to leave Deer Isle, our hostess presented us with a basket, inside of which was a ball of fluff, a kitten—a pure-bred Coon Cat. "This kind is not sold, or given away, to off-islanders," our hostess explained. Then she added, "Please take care of her."

We did. But, in time, our Coon cat, being of an independent mind, chose another owner.

There was nothing we could do about it either. Tatty, as she was named, selected our friend Mimi to be her guardian and friend, and that was the end of it. The two lived happily together for more than fifteen years. Here, is a poem Mimi wrote for her favorite cat, Tatty.

The Coon Cat of Deer Isle

She has large lamp-lit eyes, green and sometimes gold
with fur that seems to hold the cold
wind of winter when she comes in from outside.
She stands on her hind feet, upright like a little man
forgetting, we suppose, she can
not walk that way, though she sometimes tries,
a step or two and then, frustrated, cries
and resumes four-footed navigation
from room to room, seeking something
until resignation stops her quest.
Then rest is all she wants, folding herself
so neat and square in one single patch of winter sun
you'd think she'd won
it in some solar contest
the way she prizes it
and holds herself
all inside it.
We think it's her island self
showing when she's all knowing
in her perfect square of sunlit round.
Well, it's a mystery

her history
and her whole mystical being—
seeing is believing: this cat's cut from different cloth
who would rather eat mint leaves than catch a moth.

The Lore of the Cat

The Maine coon is a longhaired American cat descended from a nine-teenth-century Persian strain. Long tailed, large footed, the Maine coon is a cat of many colors, a broad-headed, big-eyed beauty whose gravely serious face is very much like a lynx's.

Maine coons usually don't like confined quarters.

Breed books often talk about the fact that the Maine coon will sleep in odd postures, and in places that don't look comfortable. It's been suggested that this goes back to the days of the square-riggers, the scruffy lodging belowdecks, but once again, this sounds mythical and not too logical. Perhaps, though, the Maine coon did experience feral life within the past century and a half, and it may be, in truth, a recently domesticated cat.

The elegance of the Maine coon is a characteristic no one ever overlooks. Its independence may come from the wild, but its noblesse oblige comes from the parlor. Steinbeck was mistaken when he in-sisted that the Maine coon was "obviously of Manx origin, and even interbreeding with tame cats they contribute taillessness. The story is that the great ancestors of the coon cats were brought by some ship's captain and that they soon went wild. But I wonder where they get their size. They are twice as big as any Manx I ever saw. Could it be that they bred with bobcat or lynx? I don't know. Nobody knows."

The ship captains coming to Maine from Ankara, Turkey, is probably accurate, but we discount the rest. And George may very well have been a Manx, but a coon cat he was not; not unless George always sat on top of his tail.

The most outrageous myth of this breed is its supposed mating with the northern lynx, or the northeastern raccoon. There's no biological possibility for it, none at all. But it's easy to see how this got started with the ancient connection between the cat and the raccoon, who do share the Felidae, if not felicitous, family tree.

The Maine coon is one of the few American-bred cats. There are only about twenty-four breeds unique to North America. At the turn of the century, it was Best in Show at Madison Square Garden, but for fifty years thereafter, the breed fell into obscurity due to the popularity of Persians and other longhaired breeds.

As an American native, the Maine coon has been subjected to some complimentary myths and some not. We make room for myths in America; we love the largest, the longest, the lowliest, the littlest, the loudest. We adhere to anything that is more, or less, than it really is. As Patricia Dale-Green, author of *Cult of the Cat,* has pointed out,

> Folklore, myth, legend and fairy-tale refer not to outer, but to inner conditions on a deep level of human experience. They do not tell of objective, but of psychic, events, and though such beliefs may not be true about the animal, they are certainly accurate in their description of what the cat meant to people, and still means to many of us today.

In Steinbeck's visit to Deer Isle, the writer, who was also a mythologist, got down to business. He quickly transformed a Persian Cat into a fictive anomaly. "Once in a while a native brings in a kitten and raises it, and it is a pleasure to him, almost an honor, but cooncats are rarely even approximately tame. You take a chance of being raked or bitten all the time."

The wildcat reputation of the Maine Coon actually contributed to the popularity of what was, at the publication of *Travels with Charley,* an obscure breed. Breeders were looking for something American, something strange, something storybooklike.

When we first visited Deer Isle in the early sixties, few people could tell us anything about the coon cat. Today, it is one of the most popular breeds around.

THE OWLCAT

Cymric

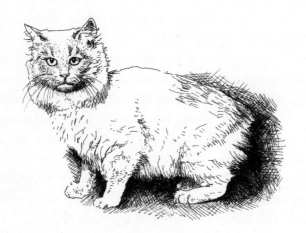

THE NINETEENTH-CENTURY NONSENSE poet Edward Lear may have just been punning when he penned his poem about the matrimony of the cat and the owl, but in point of fact, he was invoking an old Greek and Roman myth in which Athena changes into an owl and Diana transforms into a cat. Actually, the two creatures have some predatory similarities, in addition to their shared physical characteristics, and, to top it off, they are each nocturnal, and thus have the largest eyes (compared to head size) of any creature in the animal kingdom. Cats and owls, in effect, are torsos that house claws and eyes, two of the most effective arsenals of the silent hunt.

Some Native American tribes named the owl "the flying cat," while the first Europeans who came to America called burrowing owls "the winged cat."

Fred Gettings, author of *The Secret Lore of Cats,* speaks of the cat-owl connection in the following way:

> When I first heard of the Pallas Cat I thought there might lie an unexplored avenue into mythology, for Pallas was one of the titles of Athena, enshrined in the ancient mystery wisdom. What was so special about this wild cat that it should be linked by name with the esoteric tradition? Alas, the name has no such secret associations, for it is from Peter Simon Pallas, the eighteenth-century German naturalist who discovered the animal in Russia. I wonder about the magic of names, however, for the eyes of the Manul (as this cat is sometimes called) are big and directed outward in that unblinking stare associated with the owl, and when one looks frontally at such a creature one might imagine it an owl on grown legs. The point is that the attribute of Pallas Athena was an owl, and this became almost the symbol of the city to which she gave her name. Do names have a destiny, also—do names seek out creatures, rather than creatures seek out names?

Edward Lear probably said much more than he knew when he wrote "The Owl and the Pussy-Cat." Consider the poem's imagery— owl, cat, water, and moon. These archetypes revolve around the lost cyclic songs of our agrarian ancestors, whose daily and nightly blessing was given to the things that made plants grow. Owls and cats are the predators of mice—very good guardians, indeed. Plants must have water to live. The moon's recurrent calendar gives the grower time to sow and time to reap. All of these elements are interrelated.

Oddly enough, Lear must have been aware of this, for his poem is cunning, sagacious, and full of earthy wisdom, and it is also a testament to the power of myth.

Remember how it goes? The owl and the pussycat go off in a pea green boat to get married in the light of the moon.

Mythically, the boat is a symbol of unity and fecundity. Moreover, when the two animals dance upon the sand in the light of the moon, they are reenacting the glories of ancient Greek Dionysian revelry.

The poet and mythologist Robert Graves tells us that the wedding ring in the poem is yet another symbol from antiquity. It comes, incidentally, from the nose of a pig, our most venerable metaphor of earthiness.

Moreover, when the owl and the pussycat are about to be joined in wedlock, a ministerial turkey appears to perform the ceremony. Turkeys, during pagan times, were creatures of harvest and feast. In Native America they are priestly, as well, often kept as pets and rarely eaten. Overall, the turkey is the American Indian symbol of pride, goodwill, destiny, and survival. The same qualities were ascribed to this large walking bird by our European foreparents.

There are other harvest motifs in Lear's masterpiece. By marrying the cat and the owl, we are really honoring the sun and the moon. Another way of putting this is to say that, as long as the two nocturnal predators are in union, we will continue to have day and night. For, in Egyptian cosmology, the cat is the sun and the owl is the night; together they reign supreme.

Edward Lear used his own cat as an artist's model. It happens that his best friend was a bobtailed feline, whose portrait appears in some of Lear's finest drawings. With tail foreshortened and head rounded, Edward Lear's cat, Foss, looks just like a cagey old owl.

The Lore of the Cat

The Cymric (Kim-rick), another bobtailed breed, comes by this name because the Isle of Man, home of the Manx, is halfway between Ireland and Wales; and the Celtic name for Welsh is Cymric, hence the unusual-sounding name. What makes this cat different from his cousin is the long fur, which, breeders say, didn't come from Persian strains, but was bred purely from original Manx stock. Medium length, the Cymric's outer coat is shiny and smooth, but, it, too, has a thicker undercoat. This cat comes in all colors.

Lear's cat, Foss, could be either a Manx or a Cymric even though his tail is too long—about three inches from the drawings we have seen. He could be a long-tailed cat who's been robbed, bobbed, and shortened of tail. Possibly, too, a mixture of these breeds. The drawing is perhaps the most famous cat art from the nineteenth century and it offers little clue, except that the illustrator had a great imagination and, no doubt, a great cat. The drawing of the pussycat in Lear's Foss poem is certainly a bred-to-the-bone tabby. We have a feeling that Lear chose it because, among other reasons, fat tabbies do look owlish.

The Greeks linked the owl with the goddess of wisdom, Athena, who ever after gave owls the good name of knowledge. Owls nested in the buildings of the Acropolis, so there is a double significance to the reference.

In history, the owl and the cat seem to have fared well—and ill—together. Both are bound in the lore of the traditional root doctor. This mysterious physician of old was one part medical practitioner and two parts necromancer.

The spells of cats and the calls of owls both appear in Shakespeare's plays. Western literature tells us that cats are the friends of the heart; owls are the medium of the mind. The dichotomies become Ra and Apep once again.

The common aspect of the owl in folktales is usually one of portent. When the owl calls, the soul leaves. Often the cat carries on from there, acting as the intermediary between the shadows of life and death.

The owl in *Macbeth* is the "fatal bellman." The cat of eighteenth-century English poet Christopher Smart is brimming with "God's light." According to Smart, "the dexterity of the cat's defense" is the very proof of God's love.

If you have ever wondered about whether cats and owls are really alike. William Service, author of *Owl* states that they definitely are. He once had a pet screech owl and a tomcat named Claggart. The wily owl, according to Service, created a kind of amnesty in the household by using hypnotism: "I don't know what it is; it is the HEX."

This sounds as much myth as natural observation, but Service goes on to say,

In the next few hours, the two of them defined the poles of their relationship which still stand: mild aversion, indifference, and that instinctive flicker from eye to muscle, muscle to claw, or eye to gland and back to eye, or whatever and around and around, which I will call curiosity. Two rival gangs have agreed to a truce but the gunmen are a bit edgy, that's what Owl and Claggart remind me of, and their few face-to-face encounters are from the same movie.

Not what you would call an eligible marriage between a wise owl and a paunchy puss. But maybe it's just a matter of applying the right amount of hex.

THE MOUSEHOLE CAT

British Bicolor Shorthair

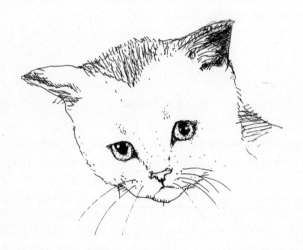

THROUGHOUT THE AGES, cats have been both thieves and the apprehenders of thieves. One of our oldest and dearest mythologies is, therefore, that of the mousehole cat. In England it is called "mowzall" and the myth expresses the primal cat-and-mouse paradigm. Visualize a fixated cat, lying down with paws folded, studying a mousehole. The cat will sit there, transfixed, all day long. Time does not matter to a cat in repose, and it matters much less to a cat in repose in front of a mousehole.

The Sanskrit word *naktacarin* is an epithet for both the cat and the thief. Mythologist M. O. Howey explains the basic dynamic of the cat's fix, and fixation:

So we see that the Cat's strange, paradoxical nature has caused her to coil herself in a circle again. She is not only the thief that cometh in the night, cloaked and hidden by its gloom. She is also the Destroyer of Thieves, the representative of the solar and lunar Eyes of Deity, before Whom "All things are naked" (Hebrews 4:13), the Exposer, the Revealer, the stark, bare Truth who had divested herself of every rag of concealment, and is the inevitable Foe of all who walk in darkness.

The cat's duality is relative to the culture of its origin. For example, in some countries the cat is the bringer of good and capturer of evil, while in others it is the bringer of evil and the capturer of good.

In the Western world, the cat has played both roles successfully. Roger Caras explains in *A Celebration of Cats* that the feline's bad rap goes back to the Buddha and to ancient Greece.

When Buddha was ill, his medicine was brought to him by a rat—some say a mouse—however, the rodent was caught by a cat and killed. So, the cat's natural inclination, for which it's usually praised, in this instance, created an unfortunate outcome. And, for this reason, the cat was the only animal not invited to the Buddha's funeral.

By killing a good rat, the poor cat got a bad name. The killing of rats and mice, says Caras, is, thus, a relative matter, culturally speaking, of course. "The priests of the Greek sun-god Apollo kept white mice as sacred animals, so one can assume that cats would not have been their favorite animal."

If one really wants to peer beneath the mythological skin of the Buddha-cat-rat topic, one ought to offer the cat a compliment. For, just as Judas delivered Jesus, the cat delivered Buddha.

But the matter centers around stealth, and Roger Caras reminds us that because the cat and the snake slip about unannounced, their hunting prowess is, itself, a matter of duality, something both good and bad.

In the world of the hunt, cats and serpents are masters. Yet, in a technological world like ours, these creatures (whether large or small, poisonous or not) are greatly mistrusted. Is this a residual remnant from the days of old?

Probably.

The serpent motif in Judeo-Christian tradition goes deep into the human psyche.

And the feline?

Caras, again: "In parts of the Roman Empire, a cat killing a bird was seen as the female element of life assaulting the male element of spirituality. But then cats have often figured in the battle of the sexes." He goes on to say that cats are a "collage of madness and myth." Of course, *our* madness, *our* myth. So, where does that leave the poor feline? As inheritors of the past, we have a certain obligation to separate the good myths from the bad. And we wonder if, sometime in the future, we'll finally break away from cattiness—our dark ruminations on the poor Felidae family.

Basically, the Neolithic dilemma is that love and hate, fear and trust, darkness and light, will always be with us, as they are, and will continue to be, the primary facets of the human imagination.

The mousehole cat is a singular theme in mythology, unless it is compared to the cat and the snake, which is another parallel theme. The politics of it is simply that we have two characters, clearly antagonistic, who are involved in an eternal, and internal, struggle to overcome one another. It is really nothing more than the high jinks of the animated pals Tom and Jerry.

Here, in pithy excerpts, we see the cat as it is—neither good nor bad—an animal possessed of itself, and, therefore, a bit unmanageable to human beings. Sometimes this unpredictable manageability shows up for the best, sometimes for the worst.

In these short meditations by Pulitzer Prize–winning playwright, William Saroyan, Michael Marseglia, and children's writer Antonia

Barber we see the mousehole cat as a killer, essayist, a friend, a fool, and a mythological force of nature.

Saroyan, on the cat as a killer:

> It was an excellent mouser, but if you've ever watched a cat toy with a mouse and finally eat it, if you've ever studied the silent terror of the wee creature, and heard its small bones being crushed in the jaws of the cat, you might very well side with the mouse. You might hate the cat. I was certainly dumbfounded that the cat could play a dirty trick like that. I didn't really imagine that the cat and mouse were playing a game, a perfectly innocent game that gave them both a great deal of pleasure, that was entirely natural and a kind of physical and spiritual calisthenics for each of them. . . . It's an unfair contest of course, but only *after* the mouse has been caught, and a wise mouse doesn't get caught.

Saroyan captures the essence of what most of us—we empathizers with the wee mousie—miss in the cat-and-mouse paradigm. To win, the mouse must not get caught, yet to succeed, the cat must capture the mouse. So the two are ever at odds and always in the embrace of their own rhythmic nature.

Michael Marseglia, on the cat as friend and fool:

> Sometime ago we were blessed with two cats. Each arrived at the household uninvited and took up residence. Since we raised birds for a living, and neither cat viewed the cage or aviary birds as prey, each cat was allowed to remain with us. Both were outside cats, but we allowed them to enter and exit the house as they wished. Early one morning, I awoke while it was still dark and opened the back door.
>
> Immediately, the two cats advanced through the open door, one of them holding a mouse between its teeth. The mouse was deposited on the floor for my inspection. Of course the mouse had no desire to be inspected, and it

ran under the china closet. There, the cats couldn't reach it, nor could I, so I got a firepoker and a broom, and, suffice to say, I eventually got the mouse back out through the front door.

Then I put the cats out and settled into a comfortable chair. A short while later the cats were back, only now the second cat had a mouse softly held in its mouth. This was deposited once again at my feet, and once more, I had to fetch the firepoker and the broom to extricate the mouse. Inconceivably, the cats came in a few minutes later—first cat with mouse in mouth—and made their usual deposit. This time, I put the cats outside, caught the mouse, freed it, locked all doors and windows, and decided to go back to bed. I was exhausted from my performance as the best mouser in the household.

Elizabeth Marshall-Thomas in *The Tribe of the Tiger* has spoken of the relationship that may, or may not, bind mice and men. Do cats really "earn their keep" by submitting mice for our approval? Or do they just enjoy the hunt? Marshall-Thomas suggests that cats seek not to please or do obeisance by placing mice indoors, but rather, they want to involve human beings with the greater pleasure of the hunt. That Michael Marseglia didn't like the early-morning game presented to him by his two felines was unthinkable to them. So their repeated efforts were an assurance, probably, that the game would go on.

Antonia Barber, on the cat as a force of nature:

And so it was that he was taken off guard as the little boat made its bid for freedom. Soothed by the sweetness of Mowzer's serenade, the Great Storm-Cat paused in his prowling and pulled back his giant cat's paw for a mere moment. Swiftly the little boat passed through the Mousehole and out into the open sea.

Then the Great Storm-Cat played with them as a cat plays with a mouse. He would let them loose for a little as they fought their way toward the fishing grounds. Then down would come his giant cat's paw in a flurry of foam and water. But he did not yet strike to sink them, for that would have spoiled his sport.

The old Cornish myth of the mousehole cat, who stops a storm and brings fish to feed the people of Mousehole, is beautifully told by Barber. However, storm cats were common fare in the British Isles and this story is not unique there. Sailors of old knew that witches were sometimes cat, sometimes kitten and they could affect the weather. The witch that worked the moon is mentioned by Shakespeare in *The Tempest*. In Ireland during a storm, cats were seized and placed in a pot and kept there until they created calm weather outside.

Witch, moon, and cat are a familiar configuration, deviling sailors all the way back to the Bible. However, the sea around the Cornish village of Mousehole was sometimes just a great pretender, blowing up a gale to keep the fishermen on their toes. In the old cat's defense, one has to admit there's no treachery in a game where the stakes are life and death. It's our common lot and whether we're animals or humans, we live by the grace of the sheathed paw of Mother Nature. To quote an Armenian proverb: "Earning our daily bread is like taking food from the tiger's mouth."

The Lore of the Cat

The classic mousehole cat is just a variation of the British bicolor shorthair cat. The fur is short and dense, the body stocky, with big round paws. The head is round, proportionate to the body. The ears, also roundish, are of medium size; and the tail is short and tapered. Colors on this cat are well defined and evenly distributed; these are cream and white, orange and white, black and white, and blue and white. A skilled mouser and fisher (he works for and with fishermen), the mousehole cat is friendly and resilient in any kind of weather.

The following prose poem by teacher Judie Eidson was written in Mousehole, Cornwall, in the inn where Dylan Thomas spent his honeymoon, and where the tale of the Mousehole Cat takes place. It says a lot about the myth of the mouse-obsessed cat, but it is also a piece of pure atmosphere, the mousehole cat come to life.

> Little Mousehole, your hedge-rowed, cow-covered, cloud-climbing hills should toss you into the sea, but your ancient gull crying, cat sunning harbour hugs you close in rough stoned embrace. I wake to early light this midsummer, calm, sea morning and pad down narrow stairs to the granite walled kitchen cozy and steam warmed. Here pilchards were once squeezed for precious oil and salted for dinner tables in Italy. I wonder if these long ago families had time to see the soft tangled green of their garden and to watch the cows summer slow munching. I think of them, and hear their far off voices, sipping tea and eating fresh Cornish strawberries on an old oak table. I sit looking out at the village at gray rock walls surprised with flowers. How lightly we touch the centuries and with so much longing, learning that this row house on Commercial Road, Mousehole (pronounced Mow-zall) was once a part of the great Pilchard works. Little Mousehole cat, sunning your flowered fur, do you know you're as literary as the wild, Welsh poet who supped at this table?

The mousehole cat comes from Egypt, where cats were first employed as guardians of the grain. In this aspect, cats have almost always been good guys, while mice have been the bad guys. Consider, too, the Native American, Amerindian, and sometimes European myth that mice nibble at the moon.

Some myths point out that cats and mice are merely dependent creatures, bound by fate to endure one another's enmity. Aesop was fond of this paradigm and he expressed it richly in his cat wife's tale, retold by Sylvia Townsend Warner. Essentially, the myth is about the man who fell in love with a cat, but once a cat always a cat, and though the goddess of love has transformed the woman, she still leaps at a mouse and eats it on her nuptial night.

In one of the well-known Noah tales, common to world mythology, the devil has created a mouse to nibble a hole in the ark; having done so, the mouse came face-to-face with a cat, who then ate him. Afterward, the hole was plugged up by a frog.

Another myth declares that Saint Francis learned to be patient while the devil's mice nibbled his robe and his toenails. Perhaps his patience might have worn thin as the mice swarmed him, but, at last, a cat leaped out of his sleeve and put an end to them. Supposedly, that cat destroyed all but two mice. These slipped into a hole, and that is why cats stare at mouseholes to this day.

THE BLACK CAT

Bombay

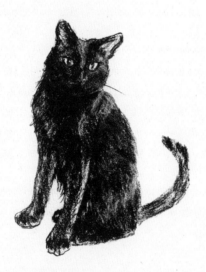

I N THE MIDI of France, the black cat is known as the *matagot,* or "magician cat." The fortunate family that takes the cat into its house receives the gift of good luck as a result. On the peninsula of Brittany, in the northwest of France, there is a similar legend called the *chat d'argent,* or "money cat." This feline is believed to serve nine owners at a time.

Throughout the rest of the world, with the exception of South America, the black cat is almost universally reviled as a harbinger of bad luck, an omen of the dark side.

Ireland, always a treasure trove of mythology, appointed the black cat as a helpmate of healers and, at the same time, a witch's familiar. Once more, this shows the pagan influence of sun and moon cycles on the human psyche.

The Irish poet W. B. Yeats liked to roam the hazel woods in search of black cats, and black cat myths. When he found such a cat, he knew the mistress or master of ancient medicine was not far away. One old-timer that Yeats interviewed at the turn of the century lived in the enchanted wood, the land of the Celtic twilight. He had seen the peculiar hedgehog named *grainne oge*. This was the odd beast who gathered ripe fallen apples by rolling his bristled back upon them, and walking off with an apple sticking to every quill.

The old worthy knew of the Celtic cats, the ones born with magic in them. "He is certain," Yeats once wrote, "that the cats, of whom there are many in the woods, have a language of their own— some kind of old Irish." The storyteller is here recorded by Yeats: "Cats were serpents, and they were made into cats at the time of some great change in the world. That is why they are hard to kill, and why it is dangerous to meddle with them. If you annoy a cat it might claw and bite you in a way that would put poison in you, and that would be the serpent's tooth."

What great change does the old storyteller refer to? Is it one of the millennial upsurges that Yeats forecasts in his most famous poem, "The Second Coming"?

> *A shape with lion body and the head of a man,*
> *A gaze blank and pitiless as the sun,*
> *Is moving its slow thighs, while all about it*
> *Reel shadows of the indignant desert birds.*

The "rough beast" is sphinxlike, slouching toward Bethlehem to be born into a world of chaos, a world in which the "falcon cannot hear the falconer," a world spinning out of control. A world in which alpha and omega are at war.

Are the Celtic cats of Irish myth merely miniatures of the slouching demon, come to wrest away the human world, and to dim the tide with the blood of sacrifice?

Once upon a time cats were revered in Europe. This was prior to the medieval witch purges. The cat's presence was then resonant with Egyptian lore of cat-headed and lion-headed goddesses. These were Bastet, the cat; Sekhmet, the lion-headed; and Ra, the sun god, who called himself Great Cat. The Egyptians worshiped the sun, the moon, and the earth, and cats were an active part of each of these worlds.

The black cat, a carrier of magic, was representative of darkness. But, owing to fur that could also turn into moonglow, or silver, the black cat was given a dual identity. Furthermore, black was the by-product of fire; fire, to the ancients was a thing of beauty, utility, and great power. All these aspects were, and are, present in the black cat.

To add to this cat's mystique, there is another myth. The Egyptians believed that each day there was a battle of the sun cat deity and the serpent of darkness. So, throughout the ages, the black cat became identified as a snakelike creature, a lunar animal. And we can also see how, in the early days of Christianity, the burned cat, the hearth cat, the night cat was thought to be devilish. After all, this was not an animal consigned to the light of day, but rather one designed to fly through the sky like the serpent with wings, the fantastical beast called the dragon.

Healer during the moon's cycles, the black cat was helpmate to the root doctors, those who gathered the dark tubers that grew by the light of the moon. When, however, the moon was full, it brought chaos and consumption, disconsolation and death. The fullness of the harvest now past, it was the moonlight itself that brought on old age. Often, then, the cat was viewed like the stages of the moon: as a kitten, white and pretty; as a young cat, full with white bloom; and, lastly, as a matriarch, gray and withered, petals fallen. Thus, the eternal female cycle.

In ancient times, cats were also the guardians of the grain. European cats, before the plague, were still beneficent spirits. They killed the rats that threatened the crop; this gave them a practical use, and as a result, the granary became their temple, and agricultural prosperity became their purpose.

The cat's mystical unity—triad of sun, moon, and earth—gave way to the garland of commerce. The pagan shrine was still there, just as in ancient days, but it was being used for a mundane rather than an arcane reason. As the European grain economies burgeoned, the cat lost her goddess status entirely, becoming now a male principled merchant. The cat, then, turned into hustler, a deal maker like the character of the morally corrupt cat in *Pinocchio,* whose friend is a wily fox.

When the plague came to Europe, the cat was cast into yet another, negative incarnation. The medieval witch, a goddess gone mad, was identified with the old serpent of darkness, Apep. She and her friend, the black cat, were the prime candidates for recrimination.

Mainly, the plague proved that the power of the goddess was dead. The new order would disown and disavow the moon goddess and the cat that went back to primordial times.

As recently as the turn of the century, however, there were still some old believers in Europe who remembered the old ways. Young W. B. Yeats found them hiding in the Celtic woodlands. He followed a doctor named Opendon, who lived in Sligo, near the "door of faeryland." Word was that, in the twilit woods, the spirits danced; and while a dog might miss such a sight, never the watchful eye of a good black cat.

Such a cat graced the hearth of Dr. Opendon, a man whose medicines were made under the cover of darkness. Bush medicines and root cures, mystically conceived, were unknown to anyone but him. Yeats tells us that he had no fixed address, for after a healing, he would fade into the candled woods with his black cat.

The black hearth cat in Ireland went back to myths of the yule log. This wood came from the sacred yew tree and it was much more than a warmer of flesh. The yew tree recalled the bygone goddesses that once reigned in the magic wood, along with the black cat, their benign familiar.

When the yew wood burned, it was called Mary Wood, or merry wood—a reference to the maiden Mary, but also to Mother Earth. Heroes, lovers, beggars, and fools knew what the wood meant, and so did bush doctors, herbsmen (once women and now men) plying their mystic trade late at night, healing those unhealed by the medical profession.

And so we have the black cat of the hearth, the cat of the night, a cat of complexity—being a little bit of Ra, the sun cat, and also

Apep, the snake. A heavy burden for so slender an animal, and yet she moves about her business with such nonchalance, such mindful grace, going first one way and then another, stepping with dew-freshened paws across the portals of time.

The Lore of the Cat

The Bombay, who resembles a small black panther, is an outcrossing of the Burmese and the black American shorthair. The enormous eyes of this cat give her a look of almost uncatlike surprise. The eyes seemingly define the face. They are gold or copper in color, and if the latter they're often designated as copper-penny eyes.

A new breed (1970s), the Bombay is considered a quiet, watchful cat who loves affection. This can be said of any feline. But the Bombay is one who, when things are going her way, purrs loudly enough to be heard in the next room. Bombays enjoy the indoors perhaps more than the outdoors, and they are noted for not liking any intrusive noises.

Visually, the cat is an artist's dream: sleek and short furred, muscular, and exceedingly well proportioned. The head, a little large for the body, is made smaller only by the dazzling eyes. A black beauty, a tranquil moon cat, a complete companion.

As the Bombay is an Asian creation, a cat harking back to a mythical model, the black panther, it would probably be well to mention the most famous of all panthery literary figures. We are thinking of course about Rudyard Kipling's Bagheera.

A quintessential cat is Bagheera, a cat in name and speech, who is of the purest of the fold. Carefully Kipling reveals him, as if uncovering a teak sculpture. And out of secrecy the great cat comes.

Within the whorls of his inky blackness, Kipling tells us, he has "panther markings showing up in certain lights like the pattern of watered silk." Noted for his cunning and his recklessness, Bagheera has a voice "as soft as wild honey dripping from a tree, and a skin softer than down."

In one of his earliest speeches to the wolf child, Mowgli, the great cat says, "I too was born among men. . . . They fed me behind iron bars from an iron pan till one night I felt that I was Bagheera—the Panther—and no man's plaything, and I broke the silly lock with one blow of my paw and came away. And because I had learned the ways of men, I became more terrible in the jungle than Shere Khan. Is it not so?"

Bagheera speaks words of wisdom, implying that the eyes of a cat will absorb what they will, and while we don't know exactly what that is, Bagheera tells us, it is power. The cat sees and stores what is known, does not forget, and becomes all the more powerful for it.

The myth of the black cat is in *The Jungle Book*. Bagheera expresses essence of cat when he informs Mowgli, "All that is in the jungle is thine." Theirs is a friendship, never sloppy, never over- stepping bounds, always framed by feline decorum: "Mowgli gentled the panther for a few minutes longer, and he lay down like a cat before the fire, his paws tucked under his breast, and his eyes half shut." Yet there is the feeling that the shadowed one will steal back into the shadows, where he can see our actions all the better. "I see you but you cannot see me," is at the heart of all cat-human friendships.

Give Kipling his due, though, for this classic novel did much to set aside the negative black cat, while restoring our faith in the cat of shadows. Bagheera is mystery without malevolence, a feline friend who can be counted on.

In Teutonic myth, the earth is bound by the Midgard Serpent, nemesis of the gods. Thor is sent to kill the creature, but it then changes into a great cat.

She is an octopus, or sea cat, whose real identity is none other than Midgard. Midgard's realm is the bottom of the sea, where the monster writhes in sea slime, just like Ursula, the octopus goddess, in Disney's animated film *The Little Mermaid*. When Ursula makes the sea boil with her rage, she recalls the cataclysmic battle, known in Teutonic myth as the Twilight of the Gods.

The serpent of darkness, in Christian lore, is, of course, the devil. Jesus, in the apocryphal Gospel Pistis Sophia, tells the Virgin Mary that "the outer darkness is a great serpent, the tail of which is in its mouth, and it is outside the whole world, and surroundeth the whole world." The serpent here is a metaphor for hell; interestingly, the great snake's accomplices are cat-faced creatures, who later become subordinate devils, but who are still cats of a kind.

THE NINE-LIVED CAT

Abyssinian

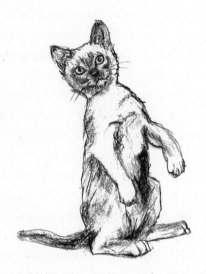

I N ARABIA, WHERE cats have been sacred since the sixth century, there springs the myth of Muhammad's cat, Muezza, the first nine-lived cat in history. It seems this blessed cat was asleep on the master's sleeve when Muhammad was obliged to go away for a brief while. Not wanting to awaken Muezza, Muhammad cut off the sleeve the cat slept on.

When the master returned, Muezza bowed in a gesture of appreciation. Muhammad then stroked Muezza three times down the length of the back, which, according to some myths, is the thing that puts cats safely on their feet when they fall.

Three is a significant number in numerology. Consider the three magi, the three wishes, the three stages of life (once a man, twice a child, as they say). Remember, too, that Muhammad's gift to Felidae was inaugurated by three strokes of the master's hand.

Moreover, as three times three equals nine, Muhammad's hand strokes multiply into greater numbers, greater powers. Mythologically speaking, a cat's life would then seem (three times three times infinity) to be endless. Many popular contemporary myths suggest that this is so. In tabloid cartoons, for instance, the cat that loses its ninth life then goes to heaven, and walks the clouds, harp in hand.

There is more to the myth of Muhammad and the cat, however. We must give some thought to the master's holy garment, that severed sleeve upon which Muezza snoozed so rapturously. What, we wonder, is the meaning of that sleeve?

A quick trip to the animated world of elementary magic gives us a clue. In Disney's masterpiece, *The Sorcerer's Apprentice,* Mickey Mouse dons his master's robe and puts on the great wizard's conical hat. The huge sleeves are cavernous, fecund with magic. Tipsy under the huge hat, Mickey struggles with a cosmic power he cannot control. As the wooden buckets of water that Mickey has conjured begin to engulf him, we see them multiply, exponentially, three times three, and three by three.

This world myth suggests that the garments of the magus are so fraught with dynamism that even off the master's body, they crackle with the energy of the universe. Thus was the robe cast off by Jesus at Golgotha, a symbol of transcendence; so, too, the so-called Shroud of Turin. Indeed, Muhammad's sleeve—the one that he severed—had its own share of potency, and was regarded thereafter as sacred. And we know from the Koran that Muhammad, in addition to being a man of wisdom, was a master of miracles—hence, a magician.

The sleeve given to the cat Muezza was a present to all cats the world over, and for all time. What was up that sleeve, no one knows, but we appreciate that it was given to Felidae, as a gift, and as a sacrament. The mythical heritage here is considerable since it conferred upon the nine-lived cat an eternity of virtue. Actions speak louder than words, and Muhammad's gesture is perfectly clear, and as if he had said, "You, my beloved cat, are a Blessed One, and shall remain in my affection forever."

The Lore of the Cat

Just as the history of the Buddha doesn't hold much of a clue as to the breed of cat that wouldn't weep at the master's funeral, so the myth of Muezza fails to tell what kind of cat it was. It is imagined, though, that Muezza might have been an Abyssinian. As a formal temple cat of ancient Egypt, this member of the Felidae clan was given a seat of oracular honor.

The rich gold-brown fur and pointed, tufted ears give the Abyssinian a lovely look, and its eyes have been called the most innocent in the world. The gaze of the Abyssinian is as euphonious and mysterious as its name.

Noted for its intelligence, this slender-bodied cat enjoys a good romp, and is equally famed for its ability to play. Overall, the cat is affectionate, soft voiced, and friendly. Its tail, long and tapered, curves back to the days of Solomon and Sheba. So legendary an animal must know things that we cannot fathom. There is an African expression for this, too: "What you don't know is wiser than you."

Numerical cat myths stretch back into antiquity. When Noah found the ark overloaded with mice, he asked Lion to solve the problem for him. Lion snorted, and out of his nostrils, first left, then right, came two cats, a female and a male. Once again, the mystical number three, for one lion and two cats are brought to the fore, as well as one lion and two magical nostrils.

In the Greek vision of hell, known as Hades, the River Styx flows in a circular fashion, making nine concentric circles.

Odin gave Freya nine worlds over which to rule.

The Egyptian pantheon consisted of nine gods.

But there is no nine more significant than the cat's best friend, woman. For it is she who gives birth on the ninth month, sharing with us the old Greek calendar of the lunar year.

THE SOLAR CAT

American Wirehair

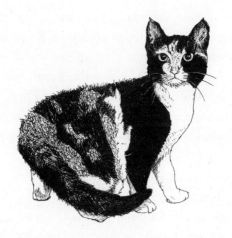

THE CONCEPT OF the solar cat, who is energized by the forces of the universe, appears in mythology throughout the world. Scientifically, it is a plausible thing, for the cat's fur is static-bearing and is, no doubt, electrically charged most of the time, Moreover, feline behaviorists have proven that cats need a certain number of solar hours each week—a large vitamin D infusion—in order to lead a normal life.

But what about the solar cat myth? Where do we see it today? Ray-O-Vac battery ads still present the logo of a fuzzy, frizzy black cat with a bolt of black lightning going through him. African American myths describe cats struck by lightning, their fur crackling with cosmic current. Black lightning, incidentally, is an occult symbol of psychic energy, the kind sought after by a conjure man, a bush doctor.

Fernand Mery author of *The Life, History and Magic of the Cat,* once said that an engineer who evaluated the electrical potential along the length of a cat's back concluded that while the cat was not exactly a generator, it was a positive storehouse of some amount of electricity. This was measured by hand strokes from the cat's head to its tail.

An actual case of cat current was discovered in a Paris TV station where a woman, seeking to calm her agitated cat by repeatedly stroking it, caused enough static electricity to scramble the images of the entire TV station.

Cartoons based on the solar, or electrical, cat were popular in the 1950s. We saw Felix, or another archetypal cat hero like Tom (of *Tom and Jerry*), whose tail, when plugged into a wall socket, turned the cat into a living lightbulb. This is nothing more, and nothing less, than the celestially powered black cat of ancient Egypt.

Behaviorists say that cats, needing a great amount of sleeping— some fourteen hours at a stretch—recharge their batteries as soon as they close their eyes. Most of us have observed the cat, who, asleep, is "shocked" awake by a dog, or by some other disturbance. Suddenly, the awakened feline is a dynamo, dancing on air—a rheostat cat, an electricat, a cat charged with stored vitality.

Philosophers have called the cat an equation for the relationship between time, space, and matter. As an envelope of fixed particles, a container of atomic structure, the cat dares to defy the physical laws of nature. It sides with MC^2 whatever limits define the cat, it is not subservient to them; the cat's energy changes shape, size, and form as needed. Here is an example: The higher, not the lower, a cat is dropped from a building (not more than four stories, not less than one), the better are its chances of survival.

We now know that the cat requires a certain amount of free fall to right itself. Imagine that the center of the cat's being is a kind of gyroscope, and that, as it falls through space, the gyroscope balances the cat's center of gravity, so that it can land safely on its feet.

Cat mythology is full of superheroes, cats who, as superbeings, perform all kinds of phenomenal stunts. However, most of these mythical characters, such as Cat Woman in *Batman,* show the cat at its best and, unbelievably, its most realistic. Hence, Cat Woman jumps off a building and lands on the street unhurt. Like the black cat that invested mythic power in her, Cat Woman is as flexible as a rubber band and as supple as a steel spring.

William Blake's famous supercat, "The Tyger," is another version of the solar cat principle, and at the same time, of Einstein's theory of relativity. Blake's cat is a living thing, a mandala of matter vibrating between spirituality and materiality. It's light, golden and liquid, and regenerates as it flows.

The reality of Tyger is eternal, and like energy, it cannot be destroyed. It can, however, swallow its tail and be reborn, as in Little Black Sambo's butter tiger, but it can never be reduced to nothingness because it is energy incarnate.

How does this relate to the common house cat, drab, humble descendant of the goddess of the Nile?

The immense harmonium of Albert Einstein, the universe, is the identical equation discovered five thousand years ago by the cat cults of Bubastis. All is movement, all is rest, says *The Egyptian Book of the Dead*.

And, therefore, All is cat.

The Lore of the Cat

The American wirehair has prickly fur, which stands out, and a bit up. The very end of each hair on this cat is bent and it looks as if the animal had been given a jolt of electricity. Extremely rare, the American wirehair is actually a mutation of the American shorthair. All the breed-accepted wirehairs of America and Canada seem to be descended from one particular cat, which was born in Verona, New York, in 1966. Fittingly, its name was Adam (Atom?).

The wirehair is a medium-size cat, well rounded and sturdy. And it really does look like that joltified animal—the frizzed fur brings a smile to the face of the observer. It comes in all colors, but it must be of the singular coat style in order to be a breed-acceptable wirehair.

Here is a cat made to order from a myth.

Mark Twain wrote about an explosive, electric cat in *Roughing*

It. The tale tells of a tabby named Tom Quartz, whose fame among the miners of Dead-House Gulch is legend.

Tom, as Ra of the Golden West, seeks the sun's favored mineral—gold. He knows the minefields better than the miners, and he lets them know when they are far afield of the glitter.

One day Tom Quartz takes a nap while the miners blast for gold. No one remembers that the poor cat is sleeping on a gunnysack by a hole charged with dynamite. The blast goes off, and the cat comes up clawing the sky, but when he touches down, he's still the same old gold-sniffing cat, just a little electrified by his experience.

Whether this is a yarn of foolery or an honored myth, Tom Quartz comes from the tradition of cats that always hold their charge.

THE GOOD LUCK CAT

Korat, Burmese, Chartreux

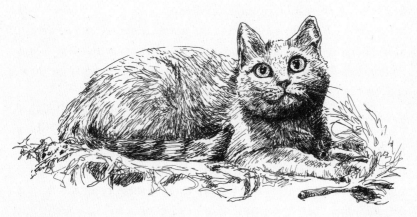

Chartreux

THE MYTHICAL *MATAGOT* from Marseilles is, by all accounts, a hungry, lucky, lonely cat with the manic disposition of a glutton. One legend says that the only way to catch a *matagot* is to lure him with a roasted chicken. Then, while the *matagot* is eating, he is captured and brought inside in a burlap sack, after which he is put into a large chest. That evening, the *matagot* is fed the first mouthful of his master's meal, and in the morning where the cat rests there will be a golden coin, the first of many feline gifts.

The folklore of the cat who confers riches is as English as it is French; in fact, the English version predates the French published myth by about one hundred years. Dick Whittington was the mayor of London in the early fifteenth century. More than that is not known about him, except that he had a cat, and the cat became famous.

The tale of Whittington's wealth, or success, seems to have been conferred by his feline friend. Whittington was an orphan, hired by one of his deceased father's creditors, and he traveled with his master to Africa. The only thing the boy owned was his cat.

That cat, according to legend, rid an African kingdom of rats. Young Dick was then given privilege as well as fortune, and he thus became a wealthy man. When he returned to London, he was a hero. In time, Dick Whittington became a prominent mayor, but his real fame rests in the canon of English folklore.

Some say this story is true to the word. And they cite evidence, too. There is, for example, the stone relief carving that was found underneath Whittington's home in Gloucester. Upon this stone there appears the image of a boy carrying a cat in his arms.

Carl Van Vechten author of *The Tiger in the House,* says that "some form of this fable exists in every language" and region, "from Moscow to Zanzibar." The oral tradition of the good luck cat is Russian, Sicilian, African, Indian, Arabian, French, Spanish, English, and American, to cite only a few. In each of these countries the cat assists a human being, perhaps, in some cases, to man's detriment, but always the cat's intent is good, and quite unlike the ambiguity extended by, say, the Cheshire Cat in *Alice's Adventures in Wonderland.*

In the Italian and East Indian version of the tale, both cat and master are swindlers of the same sort, cohorts in crime. In the Zanzibari fable, the puss is pure, the master is not. The hero wakes to find his wealth a mere vaporized dream.

The Spanish variation of the good luck cat features a friar in Mexico whose cat brings a rabbit for his master to eat at dinner. One day, an alcalde of the king's court comes to dine with the friar, whose dream is to build a great aqueduct for the village.

Seeing the cat's extraordinary wit at bringing two rabbits to table for the evening meal, the alcalde vows to secure the favor of the viceroy for the friar's water conduit.

Today, the thirty-six-arched aqueduct still stands as a testament to the good luck cat.

For those who would enjoy a modern version of the *matagot*

myth, here is Philip Greaux of St. Bart's with the tale of Boudin Creole.

I still wonder who that cat was because he sauntered into our lives uninvited, and eventually drove off our own cat, becoming, in essence, our very own legend. My father named Boudin Creole, a sort of spicy sausage made in Gua-dalupe. Boudin was wild. Apparently, no one had, in ig-norant human terms, tamed him—and no one ever did really. That first morning, Boudin came in the window by the sea and made himself right at home.

My father, who has a hot temper, caught him eating something that he shouldn't have, and, without thinking, threw Boudin out the window. Our house is two-story and built upon a hill, and although I was only seven at the time, even I knew that no cat could survive such a fall. After all, at the bottom of the hill there were jagged rocks jutting up from the sea.

However, no sooner had my father returned to his breakfast that morning than Boudin came in through the open window, and, walking over to my astonished father, buried his claws into the man's bare leg. We didn't see Boudin for a week after that, but when we did he came in through that same window with a big fat chicken in his mouth.

I thought the chicken looked a lot like one that I'd seen up at Grandfather's house (he lived a little further up the hillside), but Father was so excited by the cat's gift that he forgave him everything—and that night we had a feast, and Boudin got his new name, Boudin Creole, which means, in effect, "Hot to the touch but mighty good in-side."

Now St. Bart's isn't very big and bad news travels fast over the tropical green hills. As we sat down to eat, grandfather found his best chicken missing, along with a few of his "poussins," or chicks. So he started out to beat every dog in Anse Des Cayes, and he started a feud with his first cousin that still rages to this day.

You see, Bouzou's got a mangy dog who often frequents Grandfather's little farm, and that dog, who liked goat as well as chicken, made the perfect scapegoat (excuse the pun). Anyway, things heated up around there, but Boudin came and went as he pleased with no one suspecting anything ill of him.

Then, one afternoon I found Grandfather standing on the rock wall that borders his property. He was looking out to sea, or so I thought, and there was a rare, authentic smile on his lips (he never smiled) that ended in a deep, satisfied guffaw. I climbed barefooted onto the wall and stood beside Grandfather, and then I saw what was making him smile.

Boudin was flying around after four dogs who were abusing Grandfather's goats. These were rough-and-ready town dogs, but that cat was besting them. Finally, he drove them off and came trotting innocently over to where we were. I was never so proud of Boudin as at that moment. And Grandfather, who never has anything good to say about animals that don't lay edible eggs or produce drinkable milk, bent down and patted Boudin on the head. "I guess those dogs got a taste of the hot one," Grandfather said.

After that Boudin had the run of the family yards, and all the town dogs got the message and stayed away. Grandfather's farm seemed to prosper from this time on. Whenever a hen laid an egg it was bigger than the last and the goats when they gave milk, filled buckets. "That is one lucky cat," Grandfather said to me one day, and he meant it, too.

Years passed and I grew up and one summer Boudin disappeared. We never saw him around anymore after that, but though no one knew what became of him, I did. I was in town one afternoon when I saw an old one-eyed dog, limping on three legs, begging for food. I took one look at that face and I remembered him; he was the bully that had led the three up to Grandfather's farm. I guess he'd found just how hot Boudin Creole really was.

There is a little cairn of stones up on Grandfather's hill now and it bears the following memorial, "Hot sausage is not easy to swallow. Rest in peace, Boudin."

The Lore of the Cat

The good luck cat can be one of several breeds. The Korat, whose name loosely translates into "good fortune," is from Thailand, and is related to the *matagot,* not geographically but culturally, or rather mythically. The coat is always bluish silver rather than black; the legend is that these cats were wedding gifts to Thai brides and gifts to nobility, and their presence is recorded as far back as 1300. Soft voiced and shy, this is not a Boudin Creole, and yet it is a combative animal, especially when its territory is threatened by an outsider of the feline family. The eyes and ears are large, the body muscular, and the head has a heart shape to it.

The Burmese is another candidate for the good luck cat. Its origin is the Burmese monasteries where it was raised by monks as a temple cat. According to Roberta Altman, author of *The Quintessential Cat,* "It was believed that the soul of someone who died lived on for a period of time in the body of a sacred cat, before going on to total perfection in the next life: and that when a cat dies, he will speak to the Buddha on behalf of the owner."

A mention of the Burmese is in a book of poems published during the Ayudhya period (1350–1767). In Siam, the golden-eyed black cats were participants in religious rituals, but in Burma they were brownish in color. The body of the Burmese is muscular, with the forelegs a little longer than the hind legs. Small paws and a medium-length tail, which is pointed at the end, give this cat the look of a small chocolate panther. The coloration can also be sable, champagne, blue, platinum, or lilac, but the eyes are always gold.

The Chartreux comes from France and was bred in the monasteries of the Carthusian order near Paris. This cat was mentioned in the writings of the famous botanist Carolus Linnaeus (1707–78). In Brittany in 1931 the Legere sisters discovered a population of cats on Belle-Isle-sur-Mer and later exhibited them in France. These were true island cats from ancient stock that originated with the Carthusian monks. Why did the monks keep such cats? They were superlative hunters and their water-repellent fur enabled them to be outdoors in bad weather. Because the cat is considered legendary, this surely sounds like a *matagot*—though the Chartreux is not black, but rather slate gray.

The European shorthair is certainly a likely possibility, as this was probably the cat of Dick Whittington and also the cat of Brittany that brought good luck to the fisherfolk. The breed is especially territorial, and, though it seems to need to range around a fairly large open area, it also has a distinct family territory, of which it's most possessive. This describes Boudin Creole quite well. Part of the lucky charm is the longevity of the breed—some eighteen years or more.

The origin of the good luck cat seems to come from its survival ability, for it is the enduring cat that makes more of its kind. The cat curled up in sleep is an emblematic circle, a metaphor of life that was not lost on bestiarists of medieval Europe.

Furthermore, the enduring pattern of Stonehenge-like stones in Maidstone, in Kent, is known as Kit's Coty House. These so-called cat stones are Neolithic, primitive pieces of feline perpetuity. The cat's history, being extraordinary, portrays an animal who lived with the gods, was a god, and who lent to humans a semblance of godliness.

To stroke a cat was medicinal in old England—a touch of class, a whisper of immortality. The game of cat's cradle means Christ's cradle, or "crèche cradle"—the manger where Christ was lying, when, according to the myth, a mother cat gave birth to her kittens.

Christ as the "light of the world" is also identified with the cat in Christian imagery because the cat's eyes contain heavenly radiance.

Finally, the cat's supposed nine lives are the main reason for the belief that cats are lucky. For what other animal has extra lives with which to learn how to secure its longevity?

Certainly not the human animal. However, the cat goes around and around with the immortal fates that hold its charmed existence in abeyance, permitting it to live many lives in one.

THE CAGED CAT

Ocicat

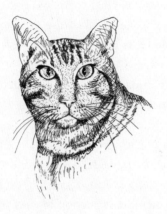

And when I mused how Time had thinned
The jungle strains within the cells,
How human hands had disciplined
Those prowling optic parallels;

I saw the generations pass
Along the reflex of a spring,
A bird had rustled in the grass,
The tab had caught it on the wing:

Behind the leap so furtive-wild
Was such ignition in the gleam,
I thought an Abyssinian child
Had cried out in the whitethroat's scream.

—E. J. Pratt

When we suspect the cat of treachery and violence, we often deliberately focus on these characteristics to the exclusion of the cat's virtues.

Some say the wildness of the cat is, and was, too much for humankind. We have only to examine our relationship with the larger cats of Felidae, the predators of big game, to achieve a clearer picture of this dynamic.

What of the big cats?

Basically, we have expelled them. We have trapped, poisoned, persecuted, banned, and jailed all of the predatory cats with whom we have ever been in close proximity. Why? Merely for being what they are, what they have always been—cats.

In the state of Florida there are an estimated 150 panthers left in the wild. And yet, prior to 1994 and not before 1924, only one person in the United States was killed by a panther in the wilderness.

What does this mean?

That the animal, as predator, has a predilection for meat, something that we also prize; and this, according to a consensus of naturalists, is what led to the near extinction of what the Native Americans called our "soft-footed brother." In that name, that gesture, is both forgiveness and receptivity to the panther; to its predation, competition with man, to even its unwillingness to be excluded from the family of life.

Today, in America, there is no warrant of brotherhood or sisterhood in the offing for the big cat. It must go, as the wild must go, and with each, something will leave us that will never return. But to the American Indian, the panther's golden hide was an intimation of immortality. It was an encapsulation of the sun.

To the European, the four-footed brother was a danger, a menace. By night, it stalked and killed cattle. Its too-quiet feet brought despair, not inspiration, because this cat could appear and disappear, could see and not be seen.

Such qualities, naturally, are also abundant in the common house cat. And our mistrust of this tabby, voiced openly by those opposed to cats, is not unlike our most ancient, subterranean fears. Symbolically, we have put the house cat in the house to keep an eye on it. The big cat we place, when it is convenient to do so, in a preserve, a reservation, a tract of land that has not been humanized.

We keep careful tabs on the Florida panther because it is endangered; but equally so because it is dangerous to humans. And what of the wildest of the wild—the big predatory cats of South America, India, Africa?

Those that are not hunted, framed by camera lens, studied, observed, and witnessed in their world are often taken to our world to beautify a place with symmetrical iron bars around it. The great poet Rainer Maria Rilke wrote of this in his poem "The Panther." Painfully, he imagines how the caged cat sees and feels his "hard-footed brother," modern man.

> *His sight from ever gazing through the bars*
> *has grown so blunt that it sees nothing more.*
> *It seems to him that thousands of bars*
> *are before him, and behind them nothing merely.*
>
> *The easy motion of his supple stride,*
> *which turns about the very smallest circle,*
> *is like a dance of strength about a center*
> *in which a mighty will stands stupefied.*
>
> *Only sometimes when the pupil's film*
> *soundlessly opens . . . then one image fills*
> *and glides through the quiet tension of the limbs*
> *into the heart and ceases and is still.*

And this is what it means to be a caught cat, a panther cat, whether large or small, that is put behind the bars of human suspicion. Will we ever let the panther cat go? Set it free? To be?

To be whatever it wishes to be, not a breed apart, but a soft-footed brother or sister?

The issue is not merely about wild animals, but all animals, domestic and wild. Cats should not need a moral contract to share our experience. We, on the other hand, ought to ask the cat's permission to enter the sanctimony of its mind.

What a world, if we were free to go, might be found there.

The Lore of the Cat

The cat that most resembles a small leopard is the ocicat, a result of a breeding experiment to produce an Abyssinian Siamese. In the 1960s a spotted kitten appeared to look a lot like an ocelot, and the breeder's daughter's vocalization, "ocicat," stuck, along with the attractive cat, who was favored to make more of his kind.

Today the breed is noted for loyalty and affection, and the unique ability to be trained. In this respect, the cat is as much Canidae as Felidae, for it doesn't mind a leash or the commands that accompany the learning of tricks. In athletics, the ocicat possesses the Abyssinian's maneuverability and speed, while also having the equanimity of the Siamese minus that inimitable voice.

Physically, the ocicat is somewhat cheetahlike: spotted, high haunched, high chested, well muscled, with a tapered, squarish muzzle and a long, slim tail. Altogether, a gorgeous cat, and a wonderful reflection of the wild.

The smallest of the predatory cats in the Americas is the jaguarundi, a native of Central and South America. This darkly furred member of Felidae has been turning up recently in southwest coastal Florida. This cat, though small at around eighteen pounds, is sometimes called the ottercat because it loves and is well adapted to water.

The jaguarundi likes grasslands, savannas, and brushlands that lie near bodies of water. Rusty brown, red, and gray are the usual colors of the cat, but there is also a color phase called "rusty spotting."

Jaguarundis may have reached the Florida peninsula from Mexico, but it's more likely that they came in through the infamous "museums" where, often during hurricanes, the wild captives escape. Talk of southeastern ottercats goes back many generations in rural parts of Florida.

The Bestiary: A Book of Beasts is a translation by T. H. White of a twelfth-century Latin bestiary. What this book says about the panther is folkloric, yet in its day, it was meant to be scientific. The cat's only enemy, the book says, is the dragon; and after eating a meal, the panther withdraws to its den to sleep for three days, after which it awakens, and belches. The belch, the bestiary explains, has the scent of spice, and all animals are drawn to this spicy fragrance with the exception of the dragon, which flees into the caves deep in the earth to escape from it.

The myth of the panther, White adds, is based upon the life of Jesus Christ, and he writes:

> The true Panther, Our Lord Jesus Christ, snatched us from the power of the Dragon-devil on descending from the heavens. He associated us with himself as sons by his incarnation, accepting all, and gave gifts to men, leading captivity captive.
>
> What Solomon pointed out about Christ is symbolized by the panther being an animal of so many colors that by the wisdom of God the Father he is the Apprehensible Spirit, the only Wise, the Manifold, the true, the Sweet, the Suitable, the Clement, the Constant, the established, the Untroubled, the Omnipotent, the All-seeing.

The breath of the panther also has religious significance. In the medieval lore of Europe, a panther's breath is the same as that of the Lord. And, as the sweetness of the panther's breath produces a calmness in all animals but the dragon, so the wisdom of Jesus brings tranquillity to the vestigial heart.

THE WORKING CAT

American Shorthair

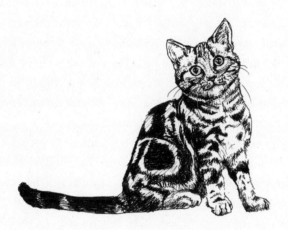

FROM THE EARLIEST of times, cats have been household guardians. However, unlike dogs, whose assignments have typically been hunting, sporting, and companionship, the house cat has been employed for basically one reason: to catch and kill mice. For this reason this breed of cat has not assumed the same importance as that of his unlikely bedfellow, the dog.

If this was traditionally the case, does it still apply today? Surveys indicate that cats are employed by us for a variety of reasons, from health care to housemate, but their age-old gift of killing vermin yet remains high on the list of human requirements.

A question that comes to mind is whether cats seem to know that their usefulness is of paramount importance in their relations with humans. Once again, the answer is positive, if not definitive. Surveys of *Cat Fancy* magazine show that cats are well aware of their status in the household and that they often become depressed when they are threatened by the loss of this status.

Enter, then, the renowned animal psychic Samantha Khury, Samantha's unusual qualifications permit her to enter the mind of the animal, and to probe that animal's feelings. In the strange case of Casey, the out-of-work cat who had become stricken with idleness, Samantha found signs of acute depression. This cat wanted his old job back. And what was that job? He was the doorman, so to speak, at his owner's restaurant. He greeted each and every person who entered through the front door. When the restaurant burned down and the owners decided not to reopen, they got on with their lives, finding new careers. But Casey just moped around the house, finally showing no interest in life at all. He was one very downhearted feline. In human terms, he might have been a potential suicide.

So Casey's owners, the Pauls, called Samantha, the psychic. And Samantha found a cause and, perhaps, a cure. Dr. Bobbie Paul was particularly surprised when she heard the news about her favorite house pet. The medical prognosis from Samantha seemed a stretch of the imagination, and she remarked, "He lost his job . . . job? What job? He is a cat. The idea of an animal needing a place to go every day, to do some kind of work, is a new concept."

However, it is not very new; in fact, it is quite old. As the guardians of the granaries, cats have held a lofty and yet very practical purpose. They have performed their duties in castles of the Old World and in the holds of ships bound for the New World. They have been ever-dutiful since the first days, and our myths proclaim this in unparalleled ways. No dog, mythically speaking, ever achieved the fame of Puss in Boots, the cavalier cat, upon whose broad leather, gold-buckled belt is hung a brace of fresh-caught mice.

Samantha had gotten her news right from the cat's mouth, or rather, from his mind: Casey wanted his old job back. No, Casey demanded his old job back. He told Samantha so, and she told Casey's family, and then there was a moment of confusion, while everyone except Samantha pondered over whether the whole thing was a hoax.

If this sounds a wee bit like a New Age fable, then accept it as such, because whatever it is, or was, it did happen, and one has only to witness the extraordinary sensitivity and accomplishment of Samantha Khury (her PBS biography on film is called *I Talk to Animals*) to understand that hers is no incidental gift, but something wonderful to behold.

Throughout her career, Samantha has uncovered the veiled secrets of cats, dogs, horses, parrots, turtles, and even elephants. What she demonstrates is that we know very little about these animals, and almost nothing about how they think and feel, and the manner in which they wish to live with their human friends.

Casey, for example, thought of himself as an indispensable maître d' at the Pauls' restaurant. While they cooked and served, Casey greeted the patrons at the door, and everything was fine until the tragic fire that closed the place down. While the family looked to other means of supporting themselves, Casey languished. They did not really notice because they were too busy with their own affairs. Normally, though, Casey would bristle with excitement while the family readied themselves for the day's work. Now, however, he lay around the house in a lackluster mood, and grew more and more despondent.

With Samantha Khury's suggestion that other work be found for Casey, the family opened their minds to this new possibility. And a few days after Samantha's healing observation, a "job" opened up for Casey. He found it himself, too.

After Samantha had given him the message that he should look for something to do, Casey went down to the public library. There, in no time at all, he became the library's official greeter, or host. Positioning himself at the front door, Casey did what came naturally to him. He smiled, he purred, he posed, he allowed himself to be petted, and he showed people in with a whisk of tail and a flash of whisker.

For a year Casey became the literary maître d' of the public library, working his usual hours and coming home a happy cat. Then the library staff ruled that animals were not welcome there, and once again Casey was out of a job.

Casey's problem came to an end when, through the help and

advice of Samantha, the Pauls found a job for Casey that could not be terminated. They started him on neighborhood visits to the homes of elderly members of the community. The end result was harmonic. Casey had found the thing he liked to do the most with the people he liked the best—those who treated him, not like a cat, but like a person. Given this respect and encouragement, Casey gave back a lot of love.

As mouser, fisher, friend, and frequently, accomplice, the cat has been indispensable as a work fellow since the days of thresh and harvest. Since then the cat as a household pet has taken its place alongside the more popular dog, but today that is changing. Because of space limitations, the human family is now increasingly favoring the house cat. And, as Casey's story shows, cats love to work. We just have to give them something to do that is commensurate with their interest and skill. Cats enjoy the pursuit of a goal as much as the pursuit of play. In fact, cat play is a kind of work to them.

David Kherdian, the Newbery Award–winning author and poet, has written many books about cats and their relationship to people. As a cat watcher, he is particularly apt at catching the cat's work-a-day posture. He suggests, perhaps rightly, that cats consider the theme of their work to be the art, or act, of watching. His poem, "The Cat" speaks of this amiable state of grace wherein the cat sees all and so becomes a part of all. Kherdian takes pleasure from, but also cognizance, for, this moment of education. For, as he says, "to see is to be."

> *Sossi sits at the top of the new-*
> *made stairs that lead to our*
> *home in the barn (finely sanded*
> *wood still to be varnished) that*
> *complement newly laid tiles on*
> *the floor beneath.*
>
> *I go and check on her, pregnant lady,*
> *but she doesn't look up at me,*
> *only wags her bushy tail, to say:*

I'm here, I hear you, I've found
my place, now leave me alone.

And so I look, too, at what she sees,
and it is good, and it is worth sitting
in front of and slowly taking in.
Through the double-doors below her
(that she faces), the hanging red
lantana plant rolls with the wind—
while the flower garden casts a final
light and color against the coming dark.

Whatever it all means or doesn't mean,
Sossi is in it—she is so completely in it
that she has become its meaning. The thing
seen and the seer have become one.

Humbly I turn and leave what is alone.

The Lore of the Cat

Casey is an American shorthair—a typical street, barn, and country cat. A bit heavier than its British cousins, the American shorthair has a longer neck and legs, and its head is also narrower. The breed was recognized as early as 1904 when a cross between the British shorthair and the common American shorthaired cat produced an all new Yankee feline.

Most experts agree that this is a cat who vibrates with pleasure when at work. According to *Cat Facts* by Marcus Schneck and Jill Caravan, "This American cat epitomizes the pioneer spirit of the nation. It is a bold, inquisitive cat with a 'working' past that needs outside spaces to roam. Always ready to do something, anything, the American Shorthair is happiest when active."

The question of the cat's work ethic occurs in cat literature of all kinds, and from all nations under the sun. It may indeed be considered the primary focus of the best cat myths—that of the cat at work; the cat who has recently accepted employment; the cat about to embark on an adventure, quest, or exalted mission.

"Puss in Boots" is of this category, and so is "The Cat Who Walked Away" by Rudyard Kipling. Mark Twain's comic tale "Dick Baker's Cat" is about a miner's pet who risks his life going to work with a man carrying dynamite.

Morris, the modern mythical tabby, the 9-Lives cat food host, was once out of work, and minutes away from euthanasia, when he landed his first big job doing a commercial.

What cats do, they do supremely well, and, we might add, seemingly without effort. Students of Zen, as noted in our chapter "The Temple Cat," have often been amused and instructed by the multiple talents of feline friends. In general, cats aren't restricted by the tasks they choose; they're unlimited.

Whatever the occupation may be—sleeping, eating, playing, working—the cat appears to put itself into an awakened mental state. Even in sleep, the cat is awake.

The cat, then, is always involved in its work. The tiny kitten shows us how naturally it can sleep in a slipper. The old tom proves that a dry birdbath in the sunshine is no less a bed than a corrugated roof, or a pile of old newspapers. Whatever the cat is doing, it is fully into the doing of it. This, consequently, is what constitutes the ease of the cat's performance, and our perennial interest in it.

The idea that when a cat is not working, it is no longer useful comes from a profound shift in human consciousness. In Europe, long after the days of cat worship were over and the fertile myths of Bubastis were but a dim memory, people still turned to the cat for sacrificial help. The societal shift here was agrarian; twelfth-century society was organized around tasks of planting and harvesting. Thus did the working cat enter as mouser, but also because of her former esteem as goddess, she was sacrificed so that a beneficial cat spirit would watch over the corn and the wheat and even the vineyard grape.

Consequently, the feline flayings and burnings associated with witches, one hundred years later, were yet in synch with cat spirit consciousness. People still believed in the power of the cat, though it was now thought to be malevolent rather than beneficent. Doubt was cast upon the poor animal by religion, fear, superstition, and the desire to place blame for the Black Plague on a common animal. Interestingly, the rat that brought the plague was excused, in a sense, by the Church because it was believed that those sinful enough to be tortured in dungeons needed to be further threatened by scourges of rats.

Today the role of the cat is far less workmanlike than it was, but cats are still believed to be charming, and that is one of their jobs. In addition, as recently as the 1960s in the United States, cats were used in post offices and transport stations to rid those environments of rats. In New Zealand, cats which were introduced to the post offices in the 1940s (in order to eat the rats that ate the mail), were listed on the civil service rolls, and were allotted a food allowance. Furthermore, maritime insurance companies in New Zealand refused to pay damages for cargo eaten by rats unless cats were proven to be on board. In the sixties, in Burma, a rat infestation in the rice fields was stopped by the deployment, by parachute, of a squadron of Singapura cats.

Obviously, the connection between cats at play and cats at work is vital to our understanding of the feline, in general. Cat out of a job seems to be a humorous conundrum, but, in truth, we find that it is not. The cat is just as devoted to us as the dog and equally aware of her need to measure up to our needs. Garfield, the sour-natured, nonworking cat of cartoon fame, has a problem—he's clearly out of work.

THE ANGELIC CAT

Turkish Angora

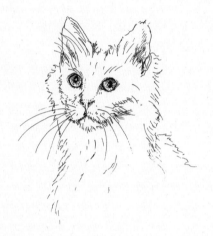

IN THE PRACTICE of magic, the function of the cat is often that of a fetish, a lucky charm, mascot, talisman or amulet." So writes Fernand Mery, who goes on to explain how important cats have been in the folklore of luck. In France and Germany, cat sacrifices included feline burials in the cornfields. Immersed in flowers, cats were tucked into a grave in the hope of affecting the spirit of the crops.

The folklore of Finland has tales of cat angels, who bear the soul of the dead to the next world. And, just as the southern United States is crowded with black cat devil tales, the Ozark Mountains contain stories of white cat saviors. In general, folklore bears out the widely held belief that white cats are as good as black cats are bad—that is, in terms of fortune. In parts of Asia, the white cat has attained a state of beatitude.

During World War II, when the Allies were trying to build supply lines through Burma, the Japanese were waging a successful propaganda war against the invading forces. No matter how much the Burmese were paid, within a few days they would abandon their work, leaving the roads unbuilt, the supply lines unfinished. Finally, an English colonel with knowledge of local customs sent his soldiers into the countryside to collect as many white cats as possible. The soldiers were also advised to paint white cats on all their military vehicles.

In a short time, with the blessing of the white cats, the Allied forces were able to get their roads built on time with the full cooperation of the Burmese people.

The white cat and its ethereal quality are reflected in nature. Albino animals have usually been treated by native people as exceptional, white being the color of the clouds, the sun, the snow.

The following story conforms to the Asian myth of the white cat that comes out of nowhere to give succor to the needy.

After Hurricane Andrew devastated South Florida, artist and friend Mariah Fox discovered a grayish cat at the door of the apartment where she was camping (her own apartment had been blown away by the 190-mile-an-hour winds) with some friends, who had also lost their home.

The cat came in the door, crying hungrily. Mariah saw immediately that the cat was pregnant. So she fed it cat food and, as she was listening to a happy song by Ziggy Marley and the Melody Makers on the radio, she decided to name the little vagabond Bright Day after the Marley song.

> *There was sunshine on the phone line*
> *And then Joy sent a note*
> *And this is what she wrote:*
> *One bright day the people got together.*

The half-starved cat walking in on a sunbeam while the song was pulsating on the boom box became the theme of the morning: guidance. The song was so cheerful and hopeful, reminding everyone that every little thing was going to be all right. Somehow, they had survived the storm, the cat had come through okay, and life, despite the awful wreckage all around, was going to continue as before.

Now, as Mariah was pregnant, too, and the need to care for something other than herself was strong in her, the white cat seemed to represent the unborn child she was carrying. The name Bright Day seemed perfect, once the cat was clean, for she wasn't a gray cat at all—she was bright white.

As the days and weeks of reconstruction passed and Miami tried to put itself back together again, after the worst hurricane in its history, Mariah and Bright Day spent a lot of time together. Mariah wrote,

> I have a spirit here to help me through this pregnancy. No, not a person-friend—a cat. I call her Bright Day. We have a little portable generator that makes a lot of noise, but at least there is electricity in our apartment (one room, six people) here in Kendall, the only room left standing in the entire broken building. The Pizza Hut down the way was destroyed and there was several hundred pounds of provolone cheese spoiling there, so the manager gave us about 50 pounds. We also have some rice in a plastic garbage barrel, and I think we are one of the only families in this area with running water. Everything looks terrible, no trees standing anywhere, just brown dirt and bombed-out buildings as if there'd been a terrible war. However, we are all well, the baby is fine, and my cat will soon have kittens, too. Looks like she's due the same day I am. Phone lines are still down. Will call as soon as the lines are up again.

A few days after we received this note, Mariah called to say that telephone service had resumed. She was breathless and had more to say about her special new cat.

> "I have to tell you that Bright Day is a perfect angel. Seriously, I think that's what she is. You know, we are living here with four Jamaican men, and I am the only woman.

It's pretty lonely being pregnant and no women around anywhere. But this cat seems to understand what I feel and she just stays around me all of the time. She is a white snowflake in a burned-out subtropical city. I feel she's here to lift my spirit, and she always manages to do so. Sometimes I cry for no reason at all, and I think it has to do with Andrew. You can't imagine what it was like. The worst was right before the winds struck and it got so quiet, but there was an awful malice in the air, like the apocalypse was coming. And, well, it did, didn't it?"

Another time she called and told us that Bright Day would go out at night and wander among the broken ficus trees by the park where there were hills around the lake.

"The frogs were singing and I looked out my window and saw Bright Day in the darkness, the only moving thing in all that black waste of fallen-down trees. She was like a fluff of cotton—no, a piece of silken silver fabric that someone had lost. And she kept appearing and reappearing like the wind was blowing her about, or as if she had wings—imagine a cat with wings, a cat angel!"

When, after some weeks, we visited Mariah, there was Bright Day, exactly as described—a kind of wonder cat, the whitest cat we had ever seen. She was positively cloudlike, snowlike, milklike, the color of the sunlight.

Bright Day liked to listen to people talk more than anything in the world. She cocked her head and really listened, trying to catch each nuance, each syllable of human speech.

Mariah was into her new apartment by this time. It was on a second floor with a balcony, and Bright Day, who had a penchant for wandering about at night, made a spectacular leap from the balcony to a tree, and from the tree to the ground. She did this so quickly it appeared that she was flying. Then she did that solitary dance on the burnt umber hills by the lake, sometimes standing on two feet and sort of waltzing for a moment or two, then leaping and running and stopping short. Her tail would flick back and forth, head turned to the stars.

Mariah, watching her with us, said: "It's like that cat is an angel. Look, she wants to fly up to heaven."

One day, shortly before her baby was due, Mariah sent us a drawing of Bright Day. Underneath it she wrote the following message.

I believe there is a silver thread attached to my soul. It's a strand of silver, strong yet delicate, stretching from my soul to the stars, if that is where I choose to travel. It's made of life, and learning, and it's held together with the people who've connected with me, past life and present. I know that Bright Day was someone to me, a person from an earlier time, perhaps. Now she's a cat—a snowy, feathery, downy white cat who is part of my silver-soul thread. She never told me who she was—I just wonder about that all the time.

The night Mariah went into labor, Bright Day did, too. She had her kittens in a brown box in the closet and Mariah had Shai, a beautiful seven-pound baby girl, at the hospital, and the family of cats and people were reunited a couple days afterward. It was a happy time for everyone. We would bring Shai to the box of kittens and she would hear them mew, three snowflakes and one dark, and Bright Day would look up at us with that inimitable cat mother's proud face, smiling so much it gave her eyes a certain slant. And that was the last we saw of her, that night. For the next day she was gone, kittens and all. She must have taken them, one at a time, to balcony, to tree, and to—wherever she felt she had to go.

The day after we looked all over for any sign of her, Mariah said without remorse,

"She came after the eve of that horrible storm, an angel sent to comfort me. She never told me who she was, and now she is only a memory and a dream. But she always knew what I was thinking and feeling, and you know what a comfort that is when you're pregnant. Now she's gone the same way she came, almost as if she was never here. But whenever I hear Ziggy's song, I think of her, and how she came out of the floating world to help rebuild and reunite our shattered lives."

The Lore of the Cat

The Turkish Angora is a slender, leggy, nicely contoured cat. Imagine white silk floating on the breeze, a gaze like the Sphinx, the voice of an angel. When we spoke to Bright Day, she responded with rapt attention, sometimes chirping, twittering like a bird. When we told her sad things, she answered with a commiserating mew.

Originally from Ankara, Turkey, this exotic breed extends far back in time. In the sixteenth century they were brought to Europe, where they helped to create the Persian, a breed that eclipsed and nearly eliminated the unfortunate Angora. In Turkey, the cat was protected as an endangered species until after World War II, when the breed made a striking comeback. In the 1960s the cat became popular in America.

This basically one-person cat comes in many colors, each and every one fragrant with poetry. The black smoke Turkish Angora, for instance, has a white coat with black tips and orange eyes. The blue smoke has a white coat with blue tips and orange eyes. The calico Turkish Angora has a white coat with black and red patches and orange eyes. The head, long and wedge shaped, is accentuated with a long regal nose; almond eyes give the cat the reputation for seeing into the human soul.

The Angora cat Bright Day had a smile that seemed to say, "It's very nice here and everything's going to be all right." In spite of her courage and apparent wisdom, she was not at all worldly. In truth, she seemed an ingenue, a debutante who had stepped upon the world's stage a bit too soon. Her innocence, too, was reflected in her mischievousness. This, we might add, frequently got her into trouble.

Bright Day was an acrobat who could leap to the height of a person's face, then drop down, tail twitching with pleasure. Noted for being an indoor cat, the Turkish Angora disdains discomfort. This was not the case with Bright Day, whose outdoor episodes always gave her a tawdry mouse gray coat. She seemed to be unaware of her condition, that her once immaculate white gown was ruined.

Never have we encountered such an unusual cat. When she went away, we somehow knew we would never see her kind again. Maybe she really was an angel, caught for a moment in a cat's coat, wondering how to get back up to heaven, just as Mariah said. In any case, we miss her.

While black cats have often been rain bearers, their color resembling the gathering of dark clouds (in Sumatra the black cat is thrown into the river by women to bring rain and fecundity to crops), the white cat is usually identified with the sun. This is an animal of combined sexes in mythology, white being seen as sunlight, or the phallus penetrating the earth, which, symbolically, is the receiving vagina.

Osiris was identified with Ra, the solar cat. Ra, in turn, was worshiped as a deity of vegetation. The moon, of course, is also catlike in world mythology. White, the moon can be female or male, depending on the culture.

In cultures where the moon is male, women fear going out into the moonlight because the moonbeams can cause pregnancy. A masculine moon is seen in the Mochica people of northern coastal Peru as a wrinkled, mustached, fanged old man.

In Danish and Celtic tales, however, a white female cat visits virgins and bestows blessings upon them. She is invariably thought to be a kind of fairy godmother. In Sicily, Saint Martha, patroness of the home, shares domestic bliss with her cat.

White cats are generally associated with freedom from burdens, suffering, privation, and punishment. They are buried in the collective unconscious as symbols of virtue, virginity, fecundity, pregnancy, and fulfillment.

THE COHORT CAT

Norwegian Forest Cat

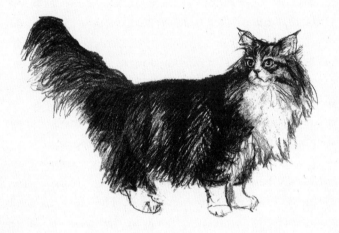

THERE'S A FUNNY kind of cat who likes to hang out with other animals who are so dissimilar from herself that, while taking on the attributes of her friends, she loses some of her—not accountability but catability, if you will.

This is the cohort cat, though she could also be called the catbird cat, when she takes up, or off, with birds, or the canine cat, when she gets too doggy for her own good. Oh, what a tangled web she weaves, this cat of sorts, this cat of sorties with animals not her kind.

Cat writer Michael Marseglia tells of the catbird cat that came to live at his aviary and farm in southwestern Florida.

A small red ball of fur emerged from under an RV and presented himself to the world. Soon it became obvious that Tiger, as we called him, was here to stay. But we didn't really encourage or feed him in the beginning since a big part of our business was raising birds—cockatiels, quakers, lovebirds, parakeets, and finches. At one point their numbers totalled more than a thousand. In addition, we had a collection of chickens of various backgrounds. A cat amongst all this varied fowl posed a very real threat.

Friends and animal lovers warned us that we had better feed the loose cat before he began taking out our birds. Until that time Tiger had survived on tiny rodents and grain, which he found in one of our chicken coops. He made his way in by shimmying down a doomed pine tree, growing out of the middle of the coop. We had roofed the coop leaving a hole for the pine, which we had no desire to kill, but which the chickens did eventually kill by supplying it with excessive quantities of nitrogen.

Tiger made his way into the coop by squeezing acrobatically between the tree trunk and the chicken wire. He made his way out the same way. The chickens were not harmed by his presence, nor were they alarmed. All he wanted was a portion of their mash and a drink of their water, so they graciously accommodated him. Seeing that Tiger didn't harm the chickens, we figured that he probably wouldn't harm the tropical birds. Then we started to coax him to the house with tuna and eventually catfood.

Today Tiger is as domesticated as any kitty born in a shoebox in the closet, and he is pushier than any domesticated cat that I know. But, back to my story: Tiger seemed to know from his earliest days with us that our chickens and our birds were off-limits to him; not the wild birds, only our caged varieties. Now one day we had a party attended by adults and children. The children wandered around the property and they got to the tropical bird cages and some of the kids opened the doors, and multitudes of finches were sent into the air.

Of course, we were quite unsettled about this. However, many of the birds hung around the yard and we were able to net them. Others, amazingly, were caught by Tiger. He would stalk his finch, get it into his mouth, gently carry it to our screened porch, and, with a muffled meow, wait for one of us to open the door. Then he would walk into the porch and drop the finch onto the floor, and we would net it. How is that for earning one's keep? I suppose Tiger managed to return twenty or thirty birds, and not one was ever harmed in the slightest way. Tiger seemed to know that the finches were something special belonging to us and they needed the most delicate delivery back into our hands.

Another kind of catbird cat is described by cat essayist Harriet Spofford. This one lived in a barn and gave birth to kittens, who, for some reason, decided to live in the henhouse. The kittens "ate with the hens, and quarreled with them for any tidbit. They curled up in the egg boxes and didn't move when the hens came to lay, and evidently had no idea that they were not chicks."

Helen M. Winslow, author of *Concerning Cats,* tells of a family of cats who hung out with a barn dog. Both cats and dog used to frequent an upstairs loft in a barn where the family kept their bantams. Strangely, the dog and his cat accomplices would steal away to the loft where they would "seat themselves around the bantam and her brood and watch them by the hour, never offering to touch the chickens except when the little things were tired and went for a nap under their mother's wings; and then some cat—first one and then another—would softly poke its paw under the hen and stir up the family, making them all run out in consternation, and keeping things lively once more. The cats didn't dream of catching the chickens."

Unusual animal relationships, partnerships, and unqualified friendships are not at all uncommon in the creature world. In our book, *The Mythology of Dogs,* the story is told of the Great Dane whose best friend was a mouse. These two comical pals charged the gossip column of the *Denver Post* with cohort news for quite some time. One might ask, with such an unusual, multidimensional relationship, did the huge Dane know that he was big and his special friend small? This question, however, is just as much a non sequitur as whether Tiger knew that her finch "friends" were edible. Animals, in any case, do not seem to recognize size in nonadversarial, which is to say, unthreatening, situations.

The Lore of the Cat

The Norwegian forest cat is a lovely, large, fluffy (it has an under- and an outercoat) feline from Scandinavia. Long clawed and large footed, she can climb rocks as well as trees. The tail is of medium length, but heavily furred, and the ruff around the neck is also heavy and thick.

This cat is known as a consummate hunter and, if given the opportunity, will hunt exclusively for her own food. Michael Marseglia's Tiger is a constant forager, one who, nonetheless, gets freshly cooked chicken every night. However, he still brings home rabbits and palmetto rats, and eats them, too.

Mythology identifies the Norwegian forest cat with the myth of Freya, the Nordic sun goddess whose chariot of fire was drawn skyward by a pair of cats. All farmers who put out milk for stray cats were blessed by Freya, who also blessed lovers and sanctified crops. Friday, in fact, is Freya's Day, and it was considered the most auspicious day for weddings. Cats, it was thought, could foretell marriages, and if a cat appeared at a wedding, it meant good tidings. So, all in all, a good feline, whose absence from the hearth meant but one thing—the cat was out hunting.

In Scandinavia, the outdoor hunter puss developed a wintry reputation for solitude and fireside meditations, and so became what is known as the butter cat. Unlike the English barn cat, whose reputation as a devourer of any dairy product was as negative as her kudos for mousing were positive, the butter cat turned into the unlikely guardian of the butter. This is the cohort cat in the extreme, but the point is, whatever the cat was, or is, it was possessed of such charm that it could be the champion of anyone, or anything, even a stick of butter.

Such a cat was also believed to scare away trolls in Lapland and from Norway to the Netherlands. The tale tells how a certain farmer always had Christmas supper with a bunch of trolls. Once, a wanderer and his pet bear came to spend the night during the feast. A troll, thinking the bear was the farmer's puss, offered the sleeping animal some food, whereupon the dreaming beast let out a fearsome growl. Now, as trolls are terrified of thunder, they all rushed out of the farmer's house—forever afraid of cats!

And that is why the cohort cat is so popular in folklore—anyone who can charm a troll into believing that it has thunder stored in its throat is a worthy friend indeed. And the friend of butter lets a little of this thunder out, too, whenever she is offered a lick of that golden treasure. But otherwise, the legend says, she will guard it as long as she lives.

The Talking Cat

Oriental Longhair

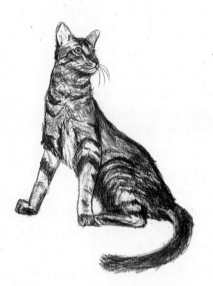

THE ANCIENT EGYPTIAN word for cat is *mau*, but the name that has stuck with us for centuries is puss, which comes from Pascht, Bast and/or Bastet. In Chinese the word for cat is also *mao*, but sometimes *miu*. In French: *minet, minoussee, mimi*. In German: *Miez, Miez-Katze*. So many lovely names for such a singular animal, and all of them applicable, onomatopoeically, to the sound that a cat makes. This implies, we think, that cats really do tell us how to say their name, by saying it for us.

In Hindustani *phis, phis* is "fish, fish"—a greeting which is still used today to call a cat, deferentially, as anyone who's ever used it should know. No recorded sound selects and stirs a cat more startlingly than "phis, phis," said in a polite and sibilant whisper. "Puss, puss," according to those experts of cat linguistics, carries some cajolery in it, and we have known cats who would rise in a rage whenever they heard this abusive talk. Generally, though, most felines disdain the cheap salute, whatever sound it is, and they'll stop and stare at you indignantly if you disturb, or alarm, them with it. "Puss, puss" is probably nothing less than some ancient, plebian flattery, for which any discerning cat feels a certain just annoyance—"Are you trying to bribe me again?"

"Meow," it would seem, is synonymous with "I see you/I recognize you." No wonder then that cats do not like repeated use of so obvious a sound when made by human beings who are impressed with their ability to reproduce it in a catlike manner. Too, the emphasis of this two-syllable greeting is important here because it conveys, depending on how it's being used, varying intensities of "seeing/greeting." For example, Siamese cats, in particular, vocalize the "ow" more pronouncedly than other breeds. Their own form of the seeing-greeting is often a long "mia-row-ow," sometimes ending in a squeak at the end of the last syllable. Decidedly, this personal use of the meow is emphatic and it may mean anything, cat linguists say, from "Hello, there, you self-centered person" to "Hello, there, you haven't fed me yet."

Some authors of cat books insist that cats, in general, refrain from speech unless it is absolutely necessary. Does this habit come from the cat or the supposed owner? Cats that don't talk are, in our opinion, not spoken to often enough, or earnestly enough—for all cats, we believe, like to talk. When cats are quiet, perhaps they have, like humans of the same disposition, nothing to say. On the other hand, or paw, as some put it, cats are really better at body language than verbal communication.

Tail talk, as any cat lover knows, is especially expressive. What is more pertinent, poetically speaking, than the wavered, lowered, flared, flowered, flaunted, flipped, tickled, trickled, and triggered tail? (Don't you wish you had one sometimes?)

Here are a few of the high signs given by cats, who use their tail as an artist's brush.

Tail straight up generally means expectant, excited, ready to enjoy, going to meet somebody or something.

Tail flat out and twitching usually suggests normalcy with a hint of irritation, depending on the frequency of the twitch: the more the twitch, the more the irritation.

Tail curled around body—peaceful, protective, do not disturb, as when a circle is drawn around as a protective cordon which says keep off, keep out.

Tail flickered at half-mast—disturbed and inquiring, or, perhaps, seeking something a little out of the ordinary, and curious about it.

Tail trembled—no doubt means hands off: "I am ready to inflict my annoyance on someone of lower status, most likely a dog."

Tail wrapped round hindquarters—fear stance offering as much coverage over sensitive region as possible.

These are but a few of the usual cat tail communiqués, and any cat person could come up with a few dozen more. The informative body language of cats has been elucidated in so many books that we do not need to get into it here. However, the notion that cats once spoke as we do is certainly worth noting. The 1960s fantasist Richard Brautigan casts a brace of malevolent yet friendly tigers in his comic novel *In Watermelon Sugar,* which includes some pertinent, as well as peripatetic, tiger talk. Here is an example.

We lived together in a shack by the river. My father raised watermelons and my mother baked bread. I was going to school. I was nine years old and having trouble with arithmetic.

One morning the tigers came in while we were eating breakfast and before my father could grab a weapon they killed him and they killed my mother. My parents didn't even have time to say anything before they were dead. I was still holding the spoon from the mush I was eating.

"Don't be afraid," one of the tigers said. "We're not going to hurt you. We don't hurt children. Just sit there where you are and we'll tell you a story."

One of the tigers started eating my mother. He bit her arm off and started chewing on it. "What kind of story would you like to hear? I know a good story about a rabbit."

"I don't want to hear a story," I said.

"OK," the tiger said, and he took a bite out of my father. I sat there for a long time with the spoon in my hand, and then I put it down.

"Those were my folks," I said, finally.

"We're sorry," one of the tigers said. "We really are."

"Yeah," the other tiger said. "We wouldn't do this if we didn't have to, if we weren't absolutely forced to. But this is the only way we can keep alive."

"We're just like you," the other tiger said. "We speak the same language you do. We think the same thoughts, but we're tigers."

Brautigan probably struck a mythic vein of gold here—the formal talk of animals in the old Buddhist texts reminds us that tigers once spoke a universal language, which all creatures, including humans, could understand. Moreover, our ancestral myths remind us that cats, large and small, have not forgotten that once-upon-a-time kingdom when humans, too, spoke "cat." Sylvia Townsend Warner, the English novelist, comments upon this in her mythic masterpiece, *The Cat's Cradle Book*:

> The difficulty, so it seems to me, would be establishing its claim (cat talk) as a serious work of scholarship. Cat is not a recognized language. How are you to convince people that what is roughly a vocabulary of mew and guttural can convey such fine shades of meaning? Scholars of Chinese, accustomed to a tonal language, might understand. But for the rest I doubt how they'd take it.

Warner's novel, a collection of interrelated short stories about cats, involves a strange young man who has learned to talk in cat. His life is further devoted to translating the best known (unto the world of the feline) myths of their version of life on earth. The narrator of the novel is a young woman who falls in love with the handsome, catlike curator of the cat barn and farm in Norfolk, England, where the translation of cat feline history is ongoing. Unfortunately, as the great work nears completion, the cat informants, who've supposedly "written" it, begin to die, one by one. Thus, their past history, their language, their codes of arcane behavior are suddenly threatened. The insistent fact remains—proof of the cats' immolation—that the word of the feline cosmos must not ever appear in print. The cat, accordingly, must reign in silence.

Perhaps cats, as visionaries, know that one day speech itself will pass from human consciousness, and we will live in telepathic bliss. Do cats—having already done away with language, as we know it— await the day? Is this what is meant by the lion lying down with the lamb? A oneness that is at once a symbiotic sharing of human thought and animal feeling? William Saroyan in the novel *Tracy's Tiger* lets his cat have the last word of silence.

This seemed a sad state of affairs so the tiger said so.

"Lune," it said.

"What do you mean?" Tracy said.

"Alune."

"I don't get it."

"Ah lune."

"What's that?"

"Lunalune."

"Doesn't mean anything."

"Ah lunalune," the tiger said patiently.

"Speak English, if you want to say something," Tracy said.

"La," the tiger said.

"That's almost French," Tracy said. "Speak English. You know I don't know French."

"Sola."

"Solar?"

"So," the tiger said.

"Don't shorten the words," Tracy said, "lengthen them so I can figure out what you're trying to say."

"S," the tiger said.

"You can talk better than that," Tracy said. "Talk or shut up."

The tiger shut up.

Whence, the rest, as the psalm says, is silence, which, in the case of the cat, always speaks louder than words.

The Lore of the Cat

Sometimes called the Mandarin, the Oriental longhair is actually only semilonghaired. In other countries—Australia and the United Kingdom—the cat is known as the Angora, the Oriental, the Javanese, and the Balinese. Elegant and striped, tigerish and talkative, the Oriental longhair seems to fit our mythical billing of a tiggery, tigery talker.

This cat has a graceful, long body, but it's also strong and muscular. The coat is fine and silky, the tail long and feathery, the face triangular, and the neck long. The eyes are almond shaped and slanted toward the nose. Colors of the tiger version of the Oriental longhair are red point, cream point, tortie point, blue-cream point, and violet-cream point. All of the above come in the lynx-point design, which is striped like a tiger. As a member of the "mystic Orient," this feline reveals herself in all kinds of ways, as mentioned above, but most notably in talking.

The talking cat is often a mischief maker in American Indian mythology. Known as the soft-footed brother, a friend from the first days of life, the cat spoke to the Osage in the following way:

> *I am the male puma who lies upon the earth.*
> *The knowledge of my courage has spread across the land.*
> *The god of day sits in the heavens.*
> *I sit close to the god of day.*

This is the sun cat, lord and friend of Father Sky. Not surprisingly, the early Incas imagined the cat nibbling the moon from full to crescent.

Old Bobcat, in the North American Indian myths, is the serious-faced joker who, according to one story, lives on the moon with a woman shaman. This seer talks too much, so she's been banished to live out her days around the cold fires of the moon. Hence Bobcat, the symbol of silence.

In European myths the tiger that walks and talks comes from many primal cultures, including East Indian (Little Black Sambo) and Irish (Pangur Bán). Legend has it that before the arrival of Saint Patrick in Ireland, all animals were fluent speakers, but he made them mute—all except the clever cats, who escaped into the Gap of the North (between Slieve Gullion and Carlingford Hills). Now, the myth continues, some of these cats were restless and went off to Egypt, where they became the objects of worship. The cats who escaped into Ulster from the south did not have to go to Egypt to have a good time, for they were long worshiped in Ireland. The deity of Fir Bolg was called Cairbre cin cait (of the cat's head) and was the enemy of the Gaulish Danann people.

Nor did the formerly talkative cat need words any longer; he thrived on the worth of his potent magic. The first cat to be mentioned by name was, in fact, the Irish puss named Pangur Bán. This cat was the friend of an eighth-century scribe who lived at the monastery of Carinthia. From the cat's mystic stare came a voice that traveled into the mind of the monk, and thus was written the poem "Pangur Bán." It is perhaps the first published cat poem in human history, and, its eight stanzas seem to say it all:

Pangur Bán

I myself and Pangur Bán,
we each have our particular skill.
His mind is fixed upon the hunt,
mine upon my chosen craft.

Peace I love beyond all fame
in diligence above my book.
    Pangur Bán is never jealous,
    holding dear his childish art.

It is never tiresome while we two
are here together in our home,
    our interest endless while we have
    something to try our skills upon.

Often, after the hard hunt,
a mouse will tangle in his net,
    while into mine there falls a rule
    of dark meaning and difficult.

He directs his pure bright eye
along the surrounding us.
    I direct my clear eye,
    weak though it is, at hard knowledge.

He takes delight in rapid action;
a mouse sticks in his sharp claw.
    Solving a dark and valued crux
    I, for my part, take delight.

However long we work together
neither one disturbs the other.
    Each enjoys his own skill
    finding pleasure for himself.

He, for his part, is the master
of his daily job of work.
    Bringing darkness into light
    is the work that I do best.

So, whether in silence or in song, the cat's words find their way into our minds, hearts, and favorite verses—that talkative cat, who doesn't have to write to make herself known throughout history.

THE PLAYFUL CAT

Seal Point Siamese

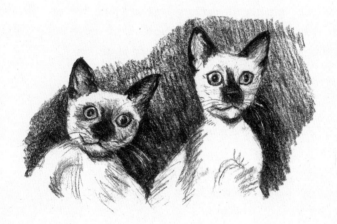

THE THING ABOUT the cat is that she seems to think that being one is so much better than not being one. Isn't this where the expression "cat's meow" comes from? The supreme feline who adores being what she is—*Felis domesticus,* the mistress of mishap. However, this entails in no small measure the ability to play, to find fun in the worst of weathers, as it were.

In the Siamese, in particular, the jade temples of the past certainly have some bearing on the cat's Oriental nature. Some experts say that the kink in the Siamese cat's past comes from the Burmese Malay cat, in which the tail is half length and often, through deformity of bone structure, curled into a knot. The so-called royal Siamese, however, has an unknotted tail, and allegedly, an unbroken past when it comes to its throne-room lineage. (More information on the Siamese kink-tailed myth is given the chapter "The Traveling Cat.") The point is, this cat has been around—up as well as down.

Although some believe the Siamese to be the smartest feline in the world (one we knew enjoyed using and flushing the toilet), no cat that we've encountered is a better example of the art of playfulness. Moreover, no cat seems to throw off despondency more gracefully than does the Siamese. It's a pleasure to watch her readjust her crown to fit the times, something we can all learn from, too.

And yet, what this cat does naturally, we seem to only sadly imitate. The nineteenth-century Japanese poet Issa (in *The Essential Haiku,* edited by Robert Hass) knows what he is talking about in describing the myth of the playful Oriental cat:

> *Having slept, the cat gets up,*
> *yawns, goes out*
> *to make love.*

> *Flopped on the fan,*
> *the big cat*
> *sleeping.*

Even in writing about the seal point, however, we are forced to imitate her artfulness. Yet there she is, teaching us by example how to live. By sleeping on a fan, the very artifice of cooling off, she is saying, "Be cool, be natural, be still." And if you think this is merely a pose, consider that most cat dilemmas ultimately end in repose. It's just that the seal point settles them more quickly than most. She shrugs, she walks away—from whatever it is that is bothering her. Even an old seal point will be aroused to play, or will discover buried humor in something that we, as humans, have overlooked.

What a healing for the human psyche the playful cat is—when life's a mess, she disdains it, then quickly plays with it. During a tropical depression in southwestern Florida, we witnessed a seventeen-year-old Siamese cat who, finding himself out of range of the house, did what came naturally.

Caught in bad weather
the old cat curls up
under the jasmine vine
and naps in the rain.

In general, the art of the playful cat is to be relaxed in the uncertainty of life, to figure a way out of mental and physical anguish. The old cat caught in the rain made a face, then did what he could to accept his surroundings—he succumbed to the fusillade of water without being washed away by it. He curled up like the vine that embraced the tree beside him, and shut out the wet. The moment he got indoors, however, he started to purr, and began to clean himself off. Yet, outside in the heavy slant of the passing storm, he curled and napped, and waited it out.

Some may not see how this behavior is playful, but it is. The acceptance of nature is artful play when we understand that all things are overcome by acceptance. By becoming one with our predicament, we are no longer opposed to it. This relaxed stance is visible in the playful, the mutually responsive, cat. Whatever happens, the playful puss is onto it, into it, and inextricably with it. How many people do you know who are capable of such equanimity?

The most playful cat we ever knew was a seal point named Soosic-poosic, which, in Armenian, means "soft, gentle."

Soosic taught us many things about how to be better people, but the best thing she passed on to us was how to live in the moment, how to enjoy each moment, as if the doing of anything was life's greatest reward, an end in itself, which of course it is, when you follow in the footsteps of a cat.

What we did not know, all during the time we had Soosic, was that she was dying of cancer. According to our vet, the cat was in constant pain from feline leukemia, and yet she never showed it or gave any indication that she wasn't in the best of health, and it was only by a chance examination that we found out. Right up until Soosic's final breath, she taught us to look at life as if it were a marvelous game. In fact, it was Soosic who taught us to play hide-and-seek, cat style. The way she played it was mysterious and magical, and quite difficult from a human point of view.

Soosic insisted that we play hide-and-seek way off in the woods behind our house. She taught us, by example, that distance did not matter. What mattered was a perfect hiding place, an undiscoverable one. We would hide far off in a field, or somewhere behind a huge moss-covered boulder, or up on the limb of a tree a good distance above the ground; wherever we went, however, that cat would find us. Wherever we went, whatever we did, Soosic found us.

We would see her coming from a long ways off, taking her time, weaving along through bracken and fern, crying while she came along delicately, tail extended high, face expectant and pleased. Invariably, when she found us, she let out a loud yowl, then came pouncing and purring, happy to have turned us up in her favorite setting, the deep woods. And this, of course, was a great time for a loving reunion. Maybe that, in truth, was the source of Soosic's pleasure in the game, as it probably is for children, too. The reunion, the discovery, the loving surprise that attends the thing found. And isn't this the true game of life, whatever game it is? To seek and to find and to be joyous over the result?

The last thing Soosic did before she died was play hide-and-seek with us. After which, exhausted, she lay on the pine needles and seemed, in her own quiet way, to merely subside. What an incalculable gift that cat gave us in her way of coming and going into and out of our lives. And still we hear her soft feet on the dry October leaves and see her coming up the steep moss-grown stony path, her little feet typing out the same simple message that we each seem to forget often enough:

> *Life's short*
> *tap it*
> *while you can.*

The Lore of the Cat

The Siamese cat probably came to America around 1890, but before that the royal family of Siam made a gift of the cat to a titled English-woman, who brought it to and bred it in England. The shorthaired variety has long been considered one of the most aristocratic members of the domestic cat family. In the 1920s, owing to the interest in the Orient, American fanciers repeatedly inbred this fine cat until the strain was weak and the animal almost became extinct.

Selective breeding returned the Siamese to its proper place in the breed pantheon, and the cat is, today, what it has always been—proud, wise, affectionate, standoffish to strangers, militantly devoted to family. Some say the Siamese is the primary "watchcat" of children, owing to Oriental myths that she once held lengthy conversations with the children of emperors. And doesn't she still do this today? What cat is more vocal than the domestic and dynastic Siamese?

The seal point is beige with light fawn on the back and almost white on the belly. The seal brown is on legs, feet, tail, mask, and ears. The gem blue eyes are most impressive when the cat is motion-less, or when "gaiting" or sighting.

There's some contention about the Siamese cat's lineage, which, at best, is lost in the jade mists of Bangkok. Experts say she may have been mixed from the royal felines of Egypt, the Annamite and the Malay cat of Burma. It's the latter who possesses the kinked tail which, some say, is the stamp of the lower caste, the street cat of Siam. No doubt, in this cat's long, eventful history, she saw all sides of the street, the high, the low, and the lowliest. She is more familiar, however, with the throne rooms of the royals and the pedestals of the priests than with the alleys of Burma and the sinkholes of Siam. Still, there's an amiable, jocular, streetwise elasticity in the Siamese that suggests fantasies of the prince and the pauper—but who really knows? An-other of those unsolved mysteries of the kinked, but not necessarily kinky, kind.

The Siamese has also been called the temple mark cat. On the backs of some "highly bred" Siamese, one sees the faint sooty shadows of a marking, a place where the cat was taken very low, in back of the neck. The old myths tell us that this mark on the pale-coated cat comes from the fire-smudged fingers of a deity.

Mythologist M. O. Howey suggests that the kink in the Siamese cat's tail is explained by a fable wherein the animal tried to remember something, and knowing it might forget, knotted its tail—or was this, once again, the doing of a deity? Although Siamese cats were around for hundreds of years before their importation to Europe and America in the nineteenth century, their origin, as we've already said, is as obscure as their mystic markings. The Burmese is certainly thought to be an ancestor.

In the Temple of Lao-Tsun in the mountains of North Burma, the last of the *kittahs,* or priests, surrounded themselves with sacred temple cats. Their belief was that after death, the human soul entered the Burmese cat, whose feet were gloved in white, whose topaz eyes turned to sapphire, and whose snowy fur reflected the skin of a golden deity.

This myth bears strong resemblance to the sun/moon cosmogony of ancient Egypt; for the cat of the sun is gold, and the cat of the moon is silver. Naturally, gold is always desirable: for as a symbol it's incorruptible and immortal. Not surprisingly, Siamese cats are among the oldest living Felidae, easily reaching over twenty, and sometimes even thirty years.

The Dilapidated Cat

American House Pet

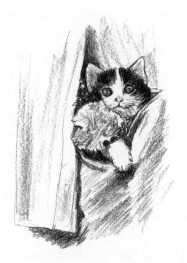

SOME CATS ARE not quite fashioned well, and there is a mythology built around this unlucky and unlikely cat, the one whose ill fortune was to have been born badly made. Writer Geoff Lalagy tells of a cat that he knew named Skrag, "the saddest cat that ever lived."

Skrag was one poor looking cat, let me tell you. She hung around our house one winter morning until we let her in and put a saucer of milk before her. A trip to the vet proved that saving Skrag's life was not a simple matter of antibiotics and nutrition. "There's something about this cat—" he said, feeling her spindly chest. Then he added, "the poor thing's dilapidated . . . not made right." That was how she got the name Skrag. She was a striped gunmetal grey with green eyes and a funny, off-kilter smile that covered all but one snaggle tooth. Among other things, Skrag had a bad case of insomnia. She sat upright wherever you put her and she rattled out this static purr that would cut on and off, as if she had no control over it. All night, Skrag stayed at the foot of our bed, weeping in one eye and making that miserable purr.

Like most cats, Skrag was a meticulous groomer. But her efforts were useless. She had the worst breath you ever smelled, and when she cleaned herself, she spread that stink all over her fur. We tried washing her, but, in a matter of hours, she'd stink again.

The saddest thing about her, though, was her disparity. All her working parts were in conflict—making her smell bad, look bad, and making everyone around her feel bad. We thought that she was unique in the Felidae category, but a little research proved that there's an entire mythology of sad-eyed, broken-down, busted luck cats.

Lalagy couldn't have hit the nail more solidly. For there is, in fact, an abundant literature and consequent mythology surrounding the dilapidated cat. One particular example of this misbegotten animal is in a poem by Pulitzer Prize–winning poet Gary Snyder:

> *I found you on a rainy morning*
> *After a typhoon*
> *In a bamboo grove at Daitoku-ji.*
> *Tiny wet rag with a*
> *Huge voice, you crawled under the fence*
> *To my hand. Left to die.*
> *I carried you home in my raincoat.*
> *"Nansen, cheese!" you'd shout an answer*
> *And come running.*
> *But you never got big.*
> *Bandy-legged bright little dwarf—*

Sometimes not eating, often coughing
Mewing bitterly at inner twinge.

Now, thin and older, you won't eat
But milk and cheese. Sitting on a pole
In the sun. Hardy with resigned
Discontent.
You just weren't made right. I saved you,
And your three-year life has been full
Of mild, steady pain.

If Skrag and Nansen are mythological archetypes, what do they represent? Life under duress, perhaps. In any case, the literary world of cats is rife with Skrags and Nansens. In Carl Van Vechten's *The Tiger in the House,* he sings the anthem of the sick cat, quoting the nineteenth-century French writer Joris-Karl Huysmans:

The fact is that this cat, thin as a hundred nails, carried his pointed head in the form of a pike's jaw and as the climax of disgrace had black lips; his fur was ashen grey, waved with rust, a vagabond's garment, with the hair dull and dry. His hairless tail was like a cord with a little tuft at the end and the skin of his belly, torn, no doubt, in a fall, hung like a fetlock of which the dirty hair swept the ground.

Huysmans goes on to say that this "low son of the race of the gutters" had a body that was a veritable "clavier of pain which resounded to each touch." Human nature, being peevish and peckish, seems to have found in such cats a reverse model of survival; the law of survival of the unfittest. Some animals, like some people, seem to thrive on ill health. Without it, they would die, possibly of boredom.

Agnes Repplier, another writer of cat sagas, speaks of an ill-arranged feline that she once knew: "He was the butt, the souffre douleur of our little society; and the inborn malignity of our natures found expression in the ridicule with which we pelted him." So, another Skrag. Well, the world is a scraggly place, indeed, when you consider that people take pleasure in finding fault with the uncomely features of animals. How reminiscent this is, too, of that classic scene in *Dumbo* when the elephant-eared boy makes fun of Dumbo's ears.

The fecundity of the cat is revered; that is, the richness of paradigm in the feline mythos. Therefore, even the unblessed cat is worthy of meter and rhyme. But what of the cat's actual fecundity? Isn't this the real reason for the Skrags of the world? The orphans of Felidae? If an archetype of ugliness exists in the cat world, and surely it does, it's not because of the cats themselves, but rather the moral failure of human beings.

What, then, of the tiers of unwanted, homeless cats? The bony and the mangy, the listless and woebegone, the nearly dead and dying, the starved and starving, the maimed and miserable. What of our refuse cats, our refused cats, our refusal of cats? What about the tens of millions of homeless felines?

Once, the cat was holy and lived only in a blaze of glory. The sistrum was softly strummed at her ear as she attended to adulatory humans, those worshipers for whom the cat was god. Long ago, the English editor of *Cat Gossip* magazine, H. C. Brooke, summed up the situation thus:

> *O Bast, look downward through the centuries*
> *And see thy children. Timorous through the streets*
> *Some crouch, the sport of every ruffian lad;*
> *Cold-blooded torturers wrench their tender limbs*
> *In name of science.*
> *Yet scarce a soul lifts a protesting voice.*

Today, however, the voice is lifted, loud and clear, and we need not look to literature to understand where Skrag came from, or why Nansen is so underfed, or even how the dilapidated cat came to be. She came to us, from us, as a gift to ourselves. And yet, we still haven't the courage to claim her as our own.

The Lore of the Cat

Skrag was, most likely, that noblest of nobody breeds, the common house pet. Gray with black stripes, small headed, awkwardly framed right down to her crooked whiskers, she was, according to author Lalagy, too "ill-made to go unnoticed."

Her tail, he mentioned, was normal "except in the middle where it was broken and had healed badly; she had white paws and the rest of her was normal, but her belly sagged like a bag of donuts."

Poor Skrag was what the poet Theodore Roethke once called a "maimed darling," a sparrow fallen from the nest of heaven. She was, on the other hand, a survivor of the first order. Nothing, Lalagy said, seemed to threaten her fatally: "In her circuitry of unconnected sinews, there was some crazy wiring that kept her alive, in spite of the hardship she'd been through. Like a creature in science fiction, she came into our lives and seemed to ask: How does it feel?"

Naturally, there is no breed specificity for the common house pet, whether she be American, Asian, or European. The only known thing about her is that we have created her, and that she is the dominant species of Bast's once great goddess clan.

Patricia Dale-Green, author of *Cult of the Cat*, talks about the dark/light psychic experience of beholding cats. She says that when we let go of our projections and see the cat for what it is, we let go of the archetypes that have bound the cat in grace, or disgrace, for ages. Cat archetypes of good and evil (with no appreciable middle ground) have formed most of humanity's fascination with felines. "The power that the cat appeared to have to attract or repel us was clearly the power of the archetype, and with the withdrawal of this 'magnet' back into ourselves, we become free."

The archetype of the broken cat is a combination of the uneven aspects of good and bad in all things—in other words, in nature itself. Dale-Green says that once we see "the cat of balance" in which all cats live, we are given a degree of detachment. This is what the Buddha called freedom from self, or personal liberation. So, to see a Skrag truly, or a measure of what made her whole, rather than disparate, is to see things as they really are.

THE DANCING CAT

Somali

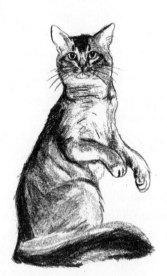

ROGER ZELAZNY AUTHOR of *To Spin Is Miracle Cat*, wrote, "Imagined cats dance at my heels." He was speaking of that mystic place in the plexus of the soul, where time whirls like an autumnal cat, eclipsing the conventions of past, present, and future. Zelazny, arguably one of our finest fantasy writers, was, like Andre Norton, Robert Heinlein, and so many others, a lover of cats.

Zelazny also knew whereof he spoke. Going to the "catyard" he called it, delving into that "vasty deep" where the world of the self begins and ends and starts anew. At the end of his own life, Roger Zelazny passed through this mortal coil surrounded by a vortex of cats—not figuratively, but literally. He was, at the last, surrounded by the seven cats of his friend and coauthor of the book *Donnerjack*, Jane Lindskold.

In the dancing cat, Zelazny observed a parable of infinity, a cat whose power was a roundness beyond riddles. In a whirl, the cat was the vasty deep; at rest, the cat became a timeless circle.

The great Japanese artists reveled in the liquidity of the cat. So did the Romans. A Roman floor mosaic discovered in Orange, France, reveals a cat in the nadir of an expanding blossom.

The sixteenth-century French essayist Montaigne discusses his cat as if, when he played with her, their identities were exchanged, she became he. Here we see the circular effect of the cat's presence:

> When my cat and I entertain each other with mutual apish tricks, as playing with a garter, who knows that I make my cat more than she makes me? Shall I conclude her to be simple, that has her time to begin or refuse to play as freely as I myself have? Nay, who knows but that it is a defect of my not understanding her language (for doubtless cats talk and reason with one another) that we agree no better? And who knows but that she pities me for being no wiser than to play with her, and laughs and censures my folly for making sport for her, when we two play together?

Author Virginia Andrews writes,

> I once saw my Somali leap from a second floor window ledge to a beech tree branch, and from there to the earth— a distance altogether of some thirty yards. One day, as I watched Amber make her customary leap, the slippery branch on which she jumped gave way, and down she tumbled.
>
> I watched, amazed, as that cloud of cumulus fur en- circled itself, until, righted, she dropped soundlessly to the grass below. I dreamed, from that moment on, of doing something like it. My mother was a gymnast and she taught me a lot about balance and grace, but her instruction was always concluded by watching our Somali cat, Amber. Day

after day, we studied her together, how she twirled and whirled, and turned to weightless fluff whenever she jumped.

Finally, when I felt I was ready, I took the dare-devil leap myself. (Of course, I didn't tell my mom about my little escapade.)

From window to tree, from tree to ground, I made my bid for immortality, jumping just like my cat, out the second-story window of my bedroom. I took the leap and, fortunately, I landed well—almost as well as Amber. Nobody saw me—unless Amber did—and that was the beauty of it. I had performed a human cat leap and no one knew but me. The confidence that one jump gave to me, growing up, is not possible to describe.

The world's a circle, Zelazny said. We are the center rider of that circle, he concluded. Observing cats brought the author to poetry and, later, to aikido.

We watched him once as he instructed some of his students in a public park in Santa Fe, New Mexico. For a man in his mid-fifties, he was light-footed and graceful, and he did these cat-quick turns, these lovely catfalls long into the leaf-falling afternoon.

Miracle cat, we thought, remembering his poem:

> *. . . our*
> *paws need licking when we*
> *pause to sort the way*
> *that cat is the quantity*
> *the maximum quantum*
> *leap of dust to blaze*
> *of day starting with eye*
> *sometimes catching language*
> *often losing words to circle*
> *and movement to utter leaves*
> *like trees to spin*
> *is miracle cat*

The self, like a dancing cat, desires to spin, to radiate beyond the prison of the flesh. Truly, when this energy is set free, it is a miracle cat, pirouetting on dancing feet beyond the confines of time and the dissolution of death.

The Lore of the Cat

A mutation of the Abyssinian, the Somali was first bred in the United States in the 1960s. With shaggy body and tail it is an obviously Oriental breed. Colors come in red with bands of chocolate brown, ruddy with bands of darker brown or black, and blue with bands of darker blue.

This cat will eagerly learn tricks and loves the freedom of the outdoors. She does not do too well as an apartment cat, some say, as she may become restless and destructive. In the outdoors, however, she is happy and resourceful, a soft bit of golden down in the green of a summer garden.

Shy by nature, the Somali is reticent about her affections and those on whom they are bestowed. While this is surely true of most cats, with the Somali it's especially true. Remember to keep her warm, though, for the Somali's not a cat of cold climes. A true Abyssinian, she takes to the warm.

Roger Zelazny's friend, Jane Lindskold, has written a short piece about her Somali, a cat named Arawn, "after the Welsh lord of the underworld, a social fellow possessed of a strong sense of justice." Jane writes, in this moving memoir of Roger and her cat, that the cat was Roger's nurse to the very end of his life.

> Arawn became Roger's devoted nursemaid; staying with him when he needed to sleep, sitting near him when chemotherapy made him weak. All through the long year until the cancer finally claimed him, Arawn never stinted on his self-imposed duties.
>
> The day Roger died, I came home to a house that would have been empty except for the cats. With me was

a close friend and, soon after, Roger's son, Trent, arrived. When Trent came in, he slung his leather jacket over the back of Goliath, a large reproduction carousel horse who dominates my living room.

As the three of us talked, Arawn leapt up onto the coffee table. Staring at me from his golden eyes, he meowed loudly, then he looked to where Roger should be sitting beside me and meowed again.

After Arawn had repeated this routine a second time, I looked at him and said softly, "I'm sorry. I can't bring Roger home."

Arawn leapt off the table, stalked over to Goliath, and vaulted three feet onto his back. Then, turning deliberately, he peed on Trent's jacket. While we gaped in disbelief, Arawn finished, leapt down, and stalked off— presumably to mourn.

I've never seen such an eloquent demonstration that cats understand what we say—and so much more than we are able to say—to them.

In the foundation-movements of the ballet, cats have been a focal point for hundreds of years. In Tchaikovsky's *Swan Lake,* for instance, the queen of the swans, when she resumes human shape, performs a "pas de chat"—a catlike leap. In *Sleeping Beauty* Puss in Boots is a main figure and so is White Cat, both characters stemming originally from the French folktales of Madame d'Aulnuy. In Sergey Prokofiev's *Peter and the Wolf,* the most popular children's ballet in America, the cat lends moral support to young Peter when he catches a wolf by the tail. The Gilbert and Sullivan opera *The Pirates of Penzance* also uses cat-walking as the pirates exit the stage toward the end, singing about their catlike tread; nor is the term "pussyfooting" to be forgotten here. All in all, the cat's dance is a myth so deeply inscribed in human consciousness that it needs no literary allusion.

Another myth of the dancing puss appears in Fred Gettings's *Secret Lore of the Cat.*

The sistrum had a variety of forms, but the most common had a cat's head (sometimes with a human face) on the upper bend of the instrument. Within the inner space were four little bars, each representing one of the four elements: it is said that the agitation of these bars represented the motion of the four elements within the material realm, by means of which form arises and is destroyed.

This, once again, is a celebration of the dancing, spinning, shape-shifting cat, who leaps into the unknown and always lands, right side up, on high ground.

THE HEALING CAT

European and American Tortoiseshell

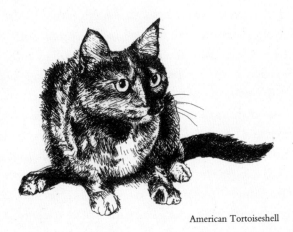

American Tortoiseshell

THE CAT OF the healing arts is the tortoiseshell, a breed whose genes are carried forth only by females. Whatever the color (from white with blood-rust spots and motes of soot, to plain white and brown), this cat is an icon of the medicine woman. In ancient times, tortoiseshells were used to cure stomach ailments. The cat, lying lengthwise on the patient's belly, was used like a hot-water bottle. Roger Caras, author of *A Celebration of Cats,* writes, "Long ago in England, the mere presence of a tortoiseshell cat could impart clairvoyant powers to the beholders, and such cats were much sought after as playmates for children." Moreover, Carl Van Vechten reminds us that "In Eastern Kansas the possession of a tortoiseshell is a surety against fire." In Japan, he says, sailors were once unwilling to put out to sea without the insurance of such a cat. The high esteem with which a ship's cat was regarded by captains of eighteenth century seagoing vessels is described by Fielding (*Voyage to Lisbon*) where such a kitten went overboard. Immediately, an alarm was given to the captain, whose bitter oaths could be heard everywhere on the deck. Then he ordered the sails slackened and sent the boatswain into the water to retrieve the cat. This man, divesting himself of jacket, breeches and shirt, leaped into the water and returned, bearing the half-drowned but still living kitten in his mouth.

The clairvoyant cat is another myth linked to the tortoiseshell. Actually, it all started with the owl and the turtle, both of which were revered by the Greeks, and later the Romans. The owl's visionary gift was wedded to the longevity of the turtle, making an indestructible seer of the two, in combination. Were tortoiseshell cats, mythologically, an amalgamation of this myth? Yes, for the cat's tortoiseshell markings and large eyes gave it the appearance of a "turtle-cat." Too, the female gender, conveying the inherent healing of motherhood, conferred a legendary status.

In addition, tortoiseshell cats may have yet another quality that sets them apart—their purr. The nature of a cat's purr has always been soothing to humans, who hear in its soft throaty rumble something of bliss and music and metaphor of mother and child reunion. So it's not surprising that a cat who is thought to be turtle-dear and owl-wise should also convey the best of velvet purrs. Ruth Wright, the owner of a tortoiseshell cat, sent us this story and poem about her own pet, whose name was Fur Purr.

Furr Purr came to us as a gift when my husband and I first met, some twenty-eight years ago. I had been the victim of a hit-and-run accident, and my husband was taking care of me. I had, at that time, a thirty pound plaster cast on my right leg, and found it impossible to sleep at night. So my husband got me a cat, a tortoiseshell cat, and I named him Fur Purr right away because of his wonderful singing voice. After getting Fur Purr, I started sleeping again, cast or no cast.

During my long recuperative time, I worried quite a bit about how my leg was healing. I had so many fractures and they were taking so long to mend. But that cat, our little Fur Purr, kept me company, always singing, all day long. And do you know where she liked to sit? On my cast, right above the knee where my bones were broken. Sometimes, I would think: Maybe, it's true what they say about tortoiseshell cats being healers. Maybe she knows where I need the most care and that's why she lies there that way.

I began imagining that my cat's purr was vibrating through that cold cast into my shattered femur, and magically knitting the fragments together. However that may sound to you, whenever my cat purred, I got the feeling that I was going to walk again. A sensation of wellness just flooded through me. Sometimes I would fall asleep listening to the water music of her purr.

Needless to say—thanks to that cat—I was on my feet after six months of recuperation. The bone healed nearly perfectly and I have been appreciative to Furr Purr ever since.

The poem that follows is my own special note of thanks to Furr Purr, who, some months after my recovery went away and did not return.

The Healing Cat

You came not to stay
but to still the pain.
This you did better than
any medicine could.

Your warm purr of love
filled the room
rumbling like
marbles of the sea—

Oh, tortoiseshell,
how you healed me!

The Lore of the Cat

The tortoiseshell cat is actually an American shorthair with mottled or splotchy fur. The coloration of Fur Purr, the author states, was an underlayment of white decorated with splashes of mocha, black, beige, and gold. A beautiful combination, perhaps even deserving of a breed, but this cat is really the descendant of the common European house cat brought to America in the 1600s.

The short-furred American variety was tested by the cold chill of a northern winter and also the rugged terrain of thorn and bracken. An all-weather cat, a cat of all seasons.

The first job of the tortoiseshell was to catch rats in the holds of ships bound for the New World. Secondly, the cat became a mouser and ratter (in farmhouse and barn), and due to the stresses of a more severe environment, it probably developed a sturdier frame and a hardier muscularity than its European cousin. The nose and face are squarish and short, with eyes and ears set apart. The face of the cat is symmetrical and in harmony with the body.

An all-terrain feline, the American shorthair withstands cold wind and raw temperatures, as well as heat and humidity. Although not noted for swimming, she can and will swim when the occasion arises, and certainly did historically, as many an account of sea voyages describe the cat going overboard, with the sturdy animal following the ship and yowling until net, rope, or first mate brought it aboard. This memory may explain why the tortoiseshell doesn't like to get wet; or you could go with the oft-cited myth that the cat was sneezed into being by the great lion of Noah's ark—a birth experience no one would forget.

The healing power of the tortoiseshell cat is, as we've said, connected to the sea. From the sea, too, comes the turtle's longevity and the modern myth of the tortoiseshell comb, which was thought, in the 1950s, to be restorative. Although very durable, it was also a soft comb, and not damaging to the hair.

Turtle amulets were one of the primary symbols of Native America, a land Indian-named Turtle Island. Europeans who came to the New World were treated to new turtle myths, which they dutifully added to their own. The basic premise of the European myth was that anything that lives so long must be blessed. The American Indians regarded the turtle as a supreme female deity, sometimes placing her together with the eagle-mother earth and father sky.

Europeans did the same thing with their pagan mythology. The turtle, the cat, and the bird were symbols of the elements of life. Hence, the woman standing on a turtle's back and holding a bird is our version of mother earth/father sky. Remember that the carryover from ancient Egypt made feminine power catlike, and stemming from the cat; the turtle was the same as the American Indian motif, also female and symbolizing the earth; and the bird—once again, female—represented the sky.

All of these visual and psychic images are compressed into the pre-Hellenic coin of woman/turtle/bird. Moreover, in time, they turned into the essential tortoiseshell cat, whose color, fur, purr, and personality were reminiscent of our ancient deities.

Nor were these unmentioned in the Bible; although the cat is not there by name, some experts say she is there by implication. However, her counterpart, the turtle of the sky, or turtledove, is present. Here was a matrimonial bird, and in the eleventh-century Christian bestiary, the turtledove is the symbol of constancy in marriage.

The theme of constancy is also the essence of what it means to be a turtle, and it is, therefore, natural that the tortoiseshell cat, our American shorthair, with those corresponding turtlelike markings, became the ultimate embodiment of all of these myths—European, Asian, and American Indian. "The flower of youth does not burn up in the turtledove, the turtle, or the cat," a medieval bestiarist once wrote. In returning to Gaea, the old European earth mother, we are learning to heal ourselves with, not a turtle-shell shaman, but a happily purring puss.

THE TEMPLE CAT

Japanese Bobtail

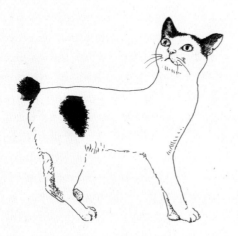

A VISITOR TO a Japanese monastery in Kyoto was surprised by the number of cats lingering at the front gate. "Why are there so many cats?" the visitor asked a nearby monk, who replied: "Cats are good. They show us the Way." Janwillem van de Wetering, author of *The Empty Mirror,* tells of a kitten he found among the pagodas and gravestones of the monastery in Kyoto where he was practicing meditation. People, he explains, often left kittens in the garden, knowing the monks wouldn't kill them because it was against their religion. By taking the kittens to a monastery, the would-be owners entrusted them to the Buddha and to the compassion of the monks. Furthermore, the depositing of cats at the monastery served a reciprocal purpose: rats, too, infested the temples.

In Japan the image of the cat adorns temples, monasteries, and shrines. In what was once Siam, cats were enshrined with members of royal houses. When a ruler was buried, his favorite cat was entombed with him. The roof of the burial chamber had holes in it, through which the cat could escape, taking the soul of the monarch with her. Such sacred cats were treated like royalty as long as they lived.

The Japanese have treasured cats in art since the earliest of times, yet perhaps one of the greatest masters of cat art was the nineteenth-century painter Hokusai. He knew well the people's love of supernatural things, and his cats fulfilled a necromancer's dream. According to legend, the color of a cat's fur indicated its powers of sorcery. Reddish cats were the most adept; white-brown-black mixes were second; and third place went to the black-and-white cat.

In general, however, Japanese artists have portrayed the feline in a variety of roles. These include the bawdy, intellectual, calculating, admiring, despairing, self-effacing, lazy, silly, sullen, and ever-endearing cat. In short, the Japanese artist seems to have caught the cat's essential nature, while the European master sought only to use the cat as a decorative item in a painting of people.

Looking at Zen cat art, the viewer is drawn to the animal's very human smile. What, the wet-brush masters seemed to ask, does the cat tell us about ourselves? What, they urged, does the cat's ineffable smile teach us about the self? The answers are many and varied, but, basically, the Zen cat is real, not imagined. Seventeenth-century paintings show cats eating, defecating, fornicating, bathing, sleeping, staring, shivering, and whining. Basho, the seventeenth-century diarist, celebrated cats in poem and painting as he made his lonely rounds on the roads of the deep north, traveling across Japan in all kinds of weather. He was, we might say, the original Dharma Bum, and his seventeen-syllable utterances are as pure a form of cat art as the world has ever known.

> *A male cat*
> *Passed through the hole*
> *In the broken hearth*
> *To meet his mistress.*

Master of the floating world, the changing, changeless void that we call the universe, Basho saw the cat as a participant, equal in all respects to human beings. As he saw it, the cat was neither divine nor profane, but a combination of the two, a quixotic mixture of each. Thus, in the poem the cat escapes from one world into another. Just as, passing through the endless rounds of birth and death, the soul travels on the solitary coil of karma.

Fernand Mery (*The Life, History and Magic of the Cat*) once wrote,

> The Japanese artists have a great deal in common with cats. They project into their creations that capriciousness of behavior and love of fantasy that, in them as in cats, is so puzzling and disconcerting. They can conceive in graphic terms a cat that is itself made of the heads of cats, whose eyes are bells, and whose bells are eyes, and many other fantasies of the same order. They patiently carve cats on their netsukes and inros. They engrave imperceptible cats on the buttons of their clothes. They give disguised cats the faces of young girls. . . . They turn a wheedling flatterer of a cat into a fiendish dragon.

Mery goes on to say that in Japanese art from the Middle Ages to the present, we may find an appreciation of the feline that is truly absent in European art, which, he remarks, "separates the greatest masters of the eighteenth century from the painters, sculptors, or engravers of the nineteenth and twentieth centuries."

The Japanese cultural attitude toward the cat is seen, and told, in a famous Nirvana picture of the Tofukuji Zen Monastery in Kyoto. Why a cat appears as a wall hanging measuring thirty-nine by twenty-six feet is explained by Dr. D. T. Suzuki, the foremost authority on Zen Buddhism. He says that the fifteenth-century painter Cho Densu promised to add the cat to his Nirvana painting if the animal would bring him the painting ingredients he needed. The cat did, and then it led him to the place where these materials could be found in abundance. Suzuki concludes, "The artist's delight was beyond measure, and to keep his word he painted the cat in his Nirvana picture, for which that cat has ever since had a nationwide reputation. Is it not a strange story? And it well illustrates the Buddhist attitude toward animals, which is also that of the Japanese people.''

There is a well-known martial arts myth, featuring a rogue's gallery of temple cats, which has been retold here by Kenji Sora, author of *The Swordsman and the Cat*.

There was once an exceptional swordsman, who was, nonetheless, unable to rid his house of a certain rat. Cleverly utilising all of the tactics of a martial artist, the rat evaded the swordsman's attempt to end its life. However, without giving up, the master summoned the aid of a neighborhood cat whose reputation for dispatching rats was unequaled.

When the black cat arrived, it rushed into the room where the rat was living and performed feats of acrobatics. In trying to subdue the rat, the cat vaulted over furniture and made itself double-jointed in squeezing under things, but still the rat vanquished the cat, and the cat bowed and left.

A second cat was summoned, this one a large tiger, who entered the room slowly, looking about for the rat. Then, seeing the rat across the room, he zeroed in on him with his eyes, creating such a burning glare that it could be felt all over the house. This cat was using a psychic force on the rat, but the rat would have none of it; walking through the electric glare of the cat's stare, it summarily threw the cat to the floor. Then they each bowed and the tiger left, humiliated.

The third cat was an average sized gray, who used a most unusual martial arts technique. This cat was a shadow-fighter and the style she employed was so nonchalant that whoever opposed her sensed that she was already defeated. In this way, and by waiting for the appropriate moment, the gray would check her aggressor's strength, find a flaw in it, and strike that flaw with merciless precision.

The gray entered the rat's room with confidence and did her usual, casual maneuver to perfection, but the rat was very, very smart. Following the gray's lead, he allowed himself to be easily beaten. Then, at the very last second, when it looked like he'd lost, he unleashed his own energy and flattened the gray with a single throw. They bowed and the female cat exited the room.

Now there was only one cat left in the neighborhood and this was a tired old master, whose inclination was not to fight any more. Most of the time, he looked like a piece of wood sitting in the sunlight. Rarely was he seen moving about, so no one paid any attention to him. Old and weary, he walked with a limp. In desperation, the swordsman called upon him at the last, and begged him to come to the house, which, by now, the rat seemed to own. No longer did he stay in just one room, but he swaggered about the whole house as if it were his.

The ancient cat, a bobtail, visited the house in a sleepy fashion, not as a competitor, but as a guest. "Ah," the rat thought, "the master has finally given up and the house is truly mine, for this oldster couldn't hurt a fly."

For several days, the rat went around so lazily that the old cat was able to sleep the whole time. One morning, however, as the rat was hauling a huge chunk of cheese to his dining area, he chanced to pass the ancient, whose eyes had not quite opened yet.

As the rat passed, the old cat's eyes flickered with interest. "Need some help?" he offered, yawning. "Sure," said the rat, "if you wouldn't mind." The old cat raised himself up and pounced on the rat, throwing him to the floor. The stunned rat couldn't get over his defeat. Bowing, he backed out of the house, never to return.

Dr. Suzuki spoke about this tale in his classic commentary, *Zen and Japanese Culture*. He quoted the master cat: "Because of the self there is the foe; when there is no self there is no foe."

Once the mind is cleansed of itself, Suzuki explained, nature can take its course, and rightful action becomes clear. The rat couldn't defeat the old master cat, whose technique consisted of no technique at all. He just waited. And then, when the time was right, he acted.

Thus the temple cat of Japan has had an influence far beyond the limitations of art.

The Lore of the Cat

The Japanese temple cat has also been called the kimono cat because it is traditionally all white with an ink spot, as it were, on its back. Any feline born with such a marking—it looks like a woman wearing a kimono—is considered sacred. The woman's shape signifies the soul of an ancestor that is within the animal. Long ago cats of this type were taken to a temple or monastery and deposited there for safe-keeping. This tradition has lived on, regardless of the cat's colors or features.

Dr. Lilian Veley, writing in *Cat Gossip* in 1910, explained that a Chinese servant took one of the kimono cats and brought it aboard a British ship, where it became the property of a British officer. The cat finally ended up at the home of a family in Putney, Vermont, where the sacred emblem of the woman in a kimono was photographed for all of America to see. What breed, if any, is the temple cat?

Authorities believe that the prototypical kimono cat was the Japanese bobtail. When the cat was born with black, red, and white coloration (tortoiseshell), the animal was considered to be good luck, a *mi-ke*, a three-color. In Japanese art, the mi-ke was often painted with one paw upraised as a gesture of goodwill. Poems celebrated her, art depicted her, and good luck charms were fashioned of her features and made into commercial items.

During and after the Second World War, mi-kes were taken

from Japan and brought to America, but the breed was still a rare thing. Unrelated to the Isle of Man Manx, the mi-ke, too, has a four- to five-inch tail. Strong and lean, the kimono, or mi-ke, is lovely to look at, as well as nice to keep, an affectionate and intelligent cat.

In Zen, the art of zazen, or sitting meditation, is sometimes taught (by example of course) by temple cats. Yet, walking meditation, alertness in movement, is no less important than the seated posture of reflection. The temple cat, as a symbol, is alert and ready for anything. However, if the cat achieves anything with regard to Zen, it is that it doesn't, consciously, achieve at all. Achievement isn't part of its world. The cat just is. This is clearly illustrated by a famous zen conversation, in which a cat bests two masters in the art of self-discovery.

> First Master (pointing to Cat): What do you call that thing
>   over there?
> Second Master: I call that thing over there a cat.
> First Master: I agree to call that thing over there, that you call
>   a cat, a cat.
> Cat: (says nothing)

THE MOTHER CAT

Turkish Van

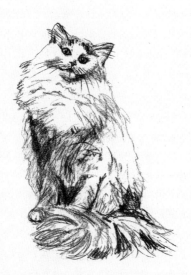

WHEN IT COMES to the policy of adoption, no animal is more accommodating, we imagine, than the mother cat. Unpredictable cat moms will adopt anything that hops, crawls, croaks, croons, or creaks—and this includes birds and mice, and, of course, men, women, and children. Michael Joseph, author of *Cat's Company,* tells of the half-Persian named Blackie, who was kind enough to adopt a young turkey as her daughter. The story is that two newly hatched turkeys hadn't a mom to look after them, and so were offered to a discerning hen, who promptly killed one, and kicked the other out of the nest. While the owner, Mrs. Lee, tried to find a suitable mother, Blackie discerned that turkeys cried just like kittens.

When Mrs. Lee next looked over at the mother cat, she saw Blackie "fast asleep with the baby turkey tucked up against her and nearly buried in her long thick fur. From that time forward Blackie seldom left it, except to catch mice, which she often brought back for her adopted daughter." Great was her confusion, however, when her newly adopted child refused her offerings, but she wouldn't be daunted. When the turkey didn't want to be bathed, kitty-style, Blackie held it down with her paw, and gave the obstinate bird a feather-dusting from stem to stern.

You might think the relationship would end when the turkey became a fully flowered bird, but this wasn't the case. Although she was no longer needed as surrogate mom, Blackie showed—even after her "daughter" had a brood of her own—that there was a deeper bond, something neither accidental nor forgettable from a feline standpoint.

Michael Joseph also remarks that cats have a very strong instinct for motherhood; this, he says, aligns them with some unlikely animal friends. Even mice, he says, have been taken into the furry fold by an amiable mother cat. Apparently, a barn cat at Beaumont, Jersey, in England, had settled in a manger with her kittens. Just above this manger was a mousehole in which there lived a baby mouse, who was motherless on account of the cat. Soon, however, the mama cat took in the baby mouse, and everything was okay until the mouse wandered off; then the cat cried until the mouse found its way back to the cat's nest. Oddly enough, the mouse suckled just like the kittens did.

Of course this scenario can work the other way around, too. Here is a noteworthy example. A fisherman living on an island in Florida fed a family of raccoons every evening. At dusk he put out fish scraps, always with a bowl of water nearby so the coons could wash the food, as is their habit. One day he observed an odd coon in the midst of the kits. This little one was unmasked, had a ringless tail, and was a bit skinnier than her brothers and sisters.

The fisherman observed that the spindly raccoon was actually a stray kitten. It amused him, though, the way the small feline washed its food, just the way the raccoons did, and how it used its front feet not as paws, but as hands—just like the raccoons.

The relationship between cats and dogs has often been maligned, parodied, and poked fun at in mythology through the ages, but the truth is that maternal bonds—if adoption is at issue—will not prevent either animal from doing its adoptive best.

Witness, for instance, the case of the Bedlington terrier pups who were taken in by a mother cat and added to her family of kittens. She raised them dutifully, catfully, treating them no differently than her own. And there is the case of the marmoset monkey who once decided to mother a kitten. They lived in a cage together, the kitten climbing like a monkey up a rope to get into the protective bars where monkey and kitty would spend all of their time, usually with the marmoset's arm relaxed around her youngster.

No example of the feline-primate friendship surpasses the story of the gorilla Koko and her adopted kitten. When the kitten died, the gorilla registered such grief that there was no question of her emotional devastation. Further, her bereavement was sustained for months.

English writer J. Symmons-Brown had a Turkish Van, whose passion in life consisted of listening to banjo music and befriending a parakeet. She writes,

> Some years ago we had a Turkish Van named Tigger, whose favorite pastime was to sit at my brother's feet while he was playing the guitar. The other favored listener was a parakeet. The bird liked to sit on the neck of the guitar, while it was being plucked. The cat sat at my brother's feet, and this went on for about a year.
>
> One day, however, my brother put the guitar on the bed and went to answer the telephone. When he came back, the parakeet was gone, but a telltale pile of feathers told the tale. Tigger had devoured her friend, but afterwards, we noticed a very different cat. She was still Tiggerish, but there was a sadness in her that went beyond the norm, we thought. After this tragic mistake, Tigger began adopting more birds as best friends. We had a number of others for her to choose from.
>
> We had a pocket parrot, a Blue-fronted Amazon, and a Maximilian parrot. Tigger was familiar with all of them,

but never really friendly to any but the parakeet. Now Tigger became the St. Francis of cats, surrounding herself with her parrot pals, and if one of them bit her tail, she paid it no mind. She inched away, out of beak range, but always near to her adopted friends.

And that was the way she chose to live her life for twelve more years; in the company of parrots. Seldom did she go out, nor did she ever leave sight of our birdcages. She was often at the foot of one of those cages, not standing but stationed, and as if on permanent guard duty.

To this day, we don't know what her intention was, but we suspect that the day she placed the parakeet in her mouth, she somehow knew that what she'd done was wrong and spent the rest of her days, thereafter, doing a curious cat penance for her sin. Whether this is true or not only Tigger could say.

This story parallels a good many old myths of cats and birds, who attempt to confound the laws of evolution. As Aesop said, "What is bred in the bone will come out in the flesh," but things often happen that prove opposite to the rule—perhaps, what rule there is, is not what we originally supposed. Between feather and fur, there is frequently a dram of compassion that may surprise us.

The eighteenth-century French fabulist La Fontaine had something to say about this in his well-known tale of the cat that ate the sparrow: They were best friends until the cat tasted sparrow's meat. Look to your friends, the author admonishes, for your best friend might be your worst enemy. On the other hand, there is the cat named Otis, who, like Tigger, adopted birds as graciously as people. He was once seen to pick up a half-frozen grackle lying in the snow, carry it home, and set it before the fire. Otis watched approvingly as his master thawed it, fed it, and released it. What can you say about such cats?

One thing is that the relationship seems not to be one-sided, for birds, on occasion, will also adopt cats. In Sir Richard Burton's short tale "The Cat and the Crow" there is evidence of animal reciprocity.

Once upon a time, a crow and a cat lived in brotherhood; and one day as they were together under a tree, behold, they spied a leopard making towards them. The crow at once flew up to the tree top; but the cat said to the crow: "O, my friend, has thou no device to save me?"

Now hard by that tree were shepherds with their dogs; so the crow flew towards them, and smote the face of the earth with his wings, cawing and crying out. Furthermore, he went up to one of the dogs and flapped his wings in his face, and went up a little way, whilst the dog ran after him, thinking to catch him.

Flying near the ground, lighting alternately, the crow tempted the dogs to tear him to pieces, all the while, leading them and their masters ever nearer to his goal. At last he bought them to the tree, under which was the leopard. And when the dogs saw the leopard they rushed upon him. The cat was saved by the craft of his friend the crow.

So, it does work both ways, the measure of adoption of the feathered and furred.

The Lore of the Cat

The Turkish Van is an Angora: white with red patches on the face and red rings on the tail. There are no other varieties except that the cat is sometimes "odd eyed"—each eye being a different color. The fur is fluffy and long and the tail is full. Generally, the cat isn't averse to wintry climates, but, like many breeds, prefers to be indoors.

The face is small and somewhat triangular. The eyes are small, closely set, and the ears are tufted and large. In order to avoid a nervous Van, one should handle it a lot from infancy on into adulthood.

The Van is naturally found around her namesake, Lake Van, in Turkey. Raised around the water, the breed has an affinity for wet stuff, and really likes to swim. An old breed, this cat has been a household pet for centuries. Her water prowess is well known in Turkey, where she's been known to swim into the harbor to greet fishing boats. Tigger, an apartment cat, had no such bodies of water available to her, but, according to Symmons-Brown, "she enjoyed climbing into a tub of cold bath water and sat there with a contented look on her face."

This breed, in the Western world, is considered new and even unaccredited. According to *The Reader's Digest Illustrated Book of Cats*:

In 1955 Laura Lushington and Sonia Halliday returned to England from a Turkish vacation with a couple of cats from the Lake Van area. Four years later, they brought home two more. The cats' white kittens with auburn markings launched the Turkish Van. It was registered in Britain in 1969 and in North America in 1985.

The mythology of the mother cat is universal. There is a Hindu sect in southern India, for instance, which professes: "God looks upon us as the mother cat looks upon her kittens: with unjudging love." Bastet, the mother figure of felinity, had the later, second name, Mut, "world mother." In Thebes, her temple was preceded by an avenue of sphinxes. Moreover, a cat-family amulet (mother cat and kittens) was worn by all newly married women and the number of kittens on the pendant matched the number of children the woman wanted.

The East Indian theme of the adoptive cat and mouse was universalized by Bidpai, whose classic fable "The Cat and the Mouse" is actually better known in Persia. Bidpai, a court jester in India, told tales pleasing to his king's ear sometime after Aesop's fables were circulated in ancient Greece. According to writer Jean Conger (*The Velvet Paw*):

The philosopher's theme, or moral as they used to say quaintly, is how foes used to become friendly and part afterwards. King Khosru Nushirvan of Persia (531–579) heard of these tales from India, and had them translated into his native tongue. From his day onward, the fables of

Bidpai have been more esteemed in Persia than the land
of their origin.

To put a cap on the cream of all of these mothering notions of
cats in the Far East and the Middle East, there is, of course, the love
of Muhammad for Muezza, his beloved cat. Here was the man who
galloped into Mecca on a snow white camel, but whose words gave
tribute to his pure white cat, Muezza (or Meuzza). Allah's Prophet,
according to myth, always waited on his cat, and though he swept
across Arabia with drawn sword, he learned patience, they say, from
a mother-teacher extraordinaire—Muezza. By cutting off his sleeve
rather than disturbing his sleeping friend when the muezzin called the
Prophet to prayer, he assured that all cats thereafter would be treated
the same, as one would treat one's own mother.

THE MARTYR CAT

Ragdoll

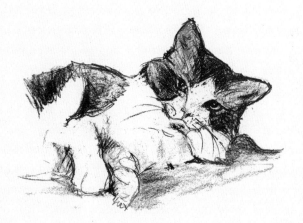

J ACK KEROUAC SPENT the last years of his life communing with his family of cats. There was one, though, for whom his affection surpassed any human bond. He loved, above the rest, a cat by the name of Tyke, a cat he held more dear than himself.

Tyke was more than the author's friend; he was a mystic companion who would, one day, quite unexpectedly, become a martyred saint to Kerouac. It was while the author was on the West Coast gathering material for the book *Big Sur* that Tyke suddenly died, throwing Kerouac into the depths of depression.

Ann Charters, author of *Kerouac: A Biography,* explains that Jack's attachment to Tyke came from something out of his own dark past. Here is how she viewed it.

Jack knew nobody could understand his feeling for his cats had always been a little crazy, that somehow he identified cats with his brother Gerard, who'd taught him to love them. Even after thirty years Tyke's death brought back painful memories of Gerard's death, but it was also a reminder of the loneliness of the life he would return to in Northport.

For his late brother, Gerard, Kerouac lamented in prose and burned candles in church, but, strangely enough, Tyke's death was akin to Kerouac's own. The final pages of *Big Sur* describe the manic rite of an author whose nightmarish vision of life is consumed with grief. Charters writes of that time,

> At dawn, nearly out of his mind, he finally found relief calling to his dead cat Tyke and hearing sudden screams that rattled through his head. He had the intuitive feeling that he was in a special state of grace if he could just hold out a little longer, and at that moment he was rewarded with a vision of the Cross that broke through his long, anguished nightmare, bringing sweet relief.

Another interesting fact is that Kerouac identified his brother Gerard with cats and crucifixes. He was obsessed with this, and with what he called his "mother's divine love." In his love of cats there is ritual, penance, and sacrifice, but it is of the most gentle kind. Here is a sample from Kerouac's *Book of Dreams*:

> The little cat I had in my hands that had such a sweet sad little funnyface with gray eyes and finally spoke to me in a pitiful little voice, like Gerard's, "J'aime pas demain" and I said "Moi too mon ange!" and felt like crying, like when I heard Ma's voice over the phone yesterday in the New York restaurant, my heart was moved just by the sound and loneliness of her voice, I'd left her alone the whole Laborday weekend and was calling at the last minute La-

borday night to say I was coming—that piteous note Gerard had, from her, and which is in my own voice when
I address little names to my cats—this kitty was an angel,
and spoke the truth—

In another chapter, Kerouac dreams of a great ghostly dog, a
huge thin giant hound that bounds across the street with Jack's cat in
his mouth: "I start to run to stop it—I know it's too late—my poor
personable kitty is gonna be dead, my little Bouncer I know it's already
inside that baskerville Beast's throat—O from where came this horrible canine of ghost??!!"

The diorama of Kerouac's psyche contains a kind of theater of
cats, who are persecuted by the author's delusions. In *Big Sur,* Kerouac
examines Tyke's passing at length, writing very tenderly of his friend.
The following is a short excerpt.

Ordinarily the death of a cat means little to most men, a
lot to fewer men, but to me, and that cat, it was exactly
and no lie and sincerely like the death of my little
brother—I loved Tyke with all my heart, who was my
baby who as a kitten just slept in the palm of my hand with
his little head hanging down, or just purring, for hours,
just as long as I held him that way, walking or sitting—He
was like a floppy fur wrap around my wrist, I just twist
him around my wrist or drape him, and he just purred and
purred and even when he got big I still held him that way,
I could even hold this big cat with my arms outstretched
right over my head and he'd just purr, he had complete
confidence in me—

Tyke's transcendent quality is also expressed by the author's
mother, Memere, who writes to him tearfully of the event of Tyke's
burial.

I buried him under the Honeysuckle vines, the corner, of
the fence. I just can't sleep or eat. I keep looking and hop-

ing to see him come through the cellar door calling "Ma Wow." I'm just plain sick and the weirdest thing happened when I buried Tyke, all the black birds I fed all Winter seemed to have known what was going on. Honest Son this is no lies. There was lots and lots of 'em flying over my head and chirping, and settling on the fence, for a whole hour after Tyke was laid to rest—I wish I had a camera at the time but God and Me knows it and saw it. Now Honey I know this is going to hurt you but I had to tell you somehow.

The so-called *Legend of Duluoz* (The life of Jack Kerouac), as packed into his twenty novels, is as revealing of us, as a culture, as it is of the road warrior, Jack Kerouac. But what it also reveals is the sorrow of a man who was not equipped to handle the dreams of his youth. His visions of destiny, fostered by high school football triumphs, were destroyed by his obsession for success, and later on, by his desire to rid himself of the agony of fame.

Tyke shows Kerouac at his most vulnerable, clutching a cat who is his past, his present, and his future. Tyke was the saint cat, the martyr cat, the cat in whose presence the author felt a moment's reprieve from the suffering of the world. However, holding Tyke, Kerouac felt the reprieve was eternal.

The Lore of the Cat

Tyke, according to Kerouac, was "a big beautiful yellow Persian, the kind they call calico." We have no definite record of Tyke's lineage, but from the descriptions given by Kerouac, Tyke was a Ragdoll. Here is why: the author says his cat is pliant beyond belief, and goes limp when picked up—"a floppy fur wrap around my wrist." He says that the cat will sleep in his hand, and when he holds him above his head, he purrs. These are indeed traits of the Ragdoll, who comes of Persian and Siamese stock.

A fairly large cat, the Ragdoll has medium-length soft fur. The head has the characteristic Siamese wedge shape and the eyes are blue. The colors include the bicolor, with pale body and dark mask, ears, and tail; the color point, which has points in seal, chocolate, or lilac; and the mitted, a color point with white paws.

The ideal owner for this cat might be a writer, but one who remains pretty much tranquil most of the time. The cat has a mild nature and doesn't like to be upset, or to be a party to upsetting things. Tyke was Kerouac's best friend, and the thought of returning home to Northport and not finding Tyke there was almost more than the author could bear.

Before leaving for California, Kerouac kissed his beloved Tyke and "instructed him to wait for me, *"Attends pour mue, kitigingoo*— But my mother said in the letter he had died the NIGHT AFTER I LEFT!"

Another feature of the Ragdoll is an uncomplaining nature. This cat, even if he'd been secretly sick before Kerouac departed, wouldn't have let on, according to many of the breed books. Ragdolls have a high tolerance for pain and they usually don't whine about life's little, or large, difficulties.

When it came out in paperback in 1963, the novel *Big Sur* sought to capitalize on Kerouac's love of cats, love of Tyke: "The King of the Beatniks—tortured, broken idol of a whole generation; great, modern sex god who just wanted to be alone with his cat." And so, we might add, the lonely cat, who himself probably died of loneliness, was the author's alter ego, his anima, his sanity in saintly robe of fur.

The martyr cat has been the subject of philosophical speculation since the first Middle English bestiaries. But before that, in their pagan worship of the corn mother cat, Europeans sacrificed cats, burying them in fields of corn to nurture their crops; these too were martyr cats.

T. H. White, author of *The Bestiary,* comments that the cat was once considered to be a metaphor for Jesus Christ. He explains that the cat, as an animal of many colors, possessed (like Jesus) many kinds of wisdom; some spiritual, some worldly, some omnipotent and all-seeing. The cat's beauty was also, White says, viewed as a correspondence with the Son of God.

However, the most important of all these aspects to the medieval monk was the martyrdom of Christ, and this, too, was compared to the sacrifice of the cat to humankind. As the word of Jesus was considered sweet, so, too, was the breath of the cat, consisting of golden mist and turning to emerald.

Although there is no specific mention of the cat in the Christian Bible, there is favorable commentary in the Talmud. In *The Gospel of the Holy Twelve* compiled by the Reverend G. J. Ouseley and published in London in 1923, there is evidence of a very old myth: "And there were in the same cave an ox and a horse and an ass, and a sheep, and beneath the manger a cat with her little ones, and there were doves, overhead, and each had its mate after its own kind."

In the same text, Jesus defends a martyred cat in the streets of a village. As it is known that the young Jesus spent time in Egypt, where cats were worshiped, there is little doubt that *The Gospel of the Holy Twelve* brings together some of the earliest Christian tales. These, according to Eleanor Booth Simmons (*Cats*), were discovered in book form in a Tibetan monastery (preserved, she believes, by the Essene order) sometime in the 1800s.

THE ARTISTIC CAT

White Persian

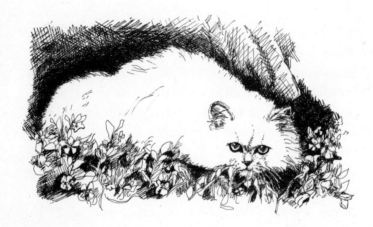

WRITERS WHO LOVE cats and write about them cannot help themselves, for no matter what they write, the cat comes in on little fog feet, forgives us, and twitches her wisp of tail. Carl Van Vechten, for example, wrote a number of books in addition to his classic *The Tiger in the House,* and all of them have little twitchy wisps of Bastet in them.

Take *The Life and Times of Peter Whiffle,* which appears to be the biography of a gentleman of the twenties. Somehow, there is a lively exchange between Mr. Whiffle, Edith Dale, and the American expatriate poet Mina Loy, out of which comes a cat-footed monologue that is better than anything Van Vechten presented in *Tiger,* and arguably some of the best cat chat we've ever seen.

The conversation between the three takes place in Florence in

1913, and mostly it's about art, but then it takes a wonderful turn into artistic cats when a gorgeous white Persian with porcelain blue eyes steps into the room. At the same time, the owner of the villa, Edith Dale, speaks about how art must be subservient to cat. That is how the curious conversation begins, but soon it becomes a lecture, not only on art but the art of living, as Ms. Dale skims across the mythology of cats, covering the gloss and the dross of what's been thought and said over the centuries. It has all of the largesse, disdain, and hauteur of the White Persian who inspired it.

> The great artists put themselves into their work; the cat never does. Men like Stieglitz and de Meyer put themselves into their cameras, that is why their photographs are wonderful, but the cat never puts himself into a camera. The great conquerors put themselves into their actions; the cat never does. Lovers put themselves into the selves of their loved ones, seeking identity; the cat never does. Mystics try to lose themselves in union with their gods; the cat never does. Musicians put themselves into their instruments; the cat never does. Indian men, working in the ground, put themselves in the earth, in order to get themselves back in the forms of wheat or maize to nourish their bodies; the cat never does. Navajo women, when they weave blankets, go so completely into the blanket while they are working on it, that they always leave a path in the weaving that comes out at the last corner for their souls to get out of the blanket; otherwise they would be imprisoned in it. The cat never does things like this!
>
> So every one really centres his self somewhere outside of himself; every one gets out of his body. The cat never does. Every one has a false centre. Only the cat—the feline—has a true centredness inside himself. Dogs and other animals centre themselves in people and are therefore open to influence. The cat stays at home inside his body and can never be influenced.
>
> Every one has always worked magic through these

false centres—doing things to himself—seeking outlets, seeking expression, seeking power, all of which are only temporarily satisfactory like a movement of the bowels, which is all it amounts to on the psychic plane. The cat is magic, is himself, is power. The cat knows how to live, staying as he does inside his own body, for that is the only place where he can live! That is the only place where he can experience being here and now.

Of course, all the false-centred people have a kind of magic power, for any centredness is power, but it doesn't last and it doesn't satisfy them. Art has been the greatest deceiver of all—the better the art, the greater the deception. It isn't necessary to objectify or express experience. What IS necessary IS to be. The cat knows this. Maybe, that is why the cat has been an object of worship; maybe the ancients felt intuitively that the cat had the truth in him.

Do you see where these reflections lead? The whole world is wildly pursuing a mirage; only the cat is at home, so to speak.

Actors understand this. They only get a sense of reality when they throw themselves into a part . . . a false centre.

The cat understands pure being, which is all we need to know and which it takes a lifetime to learn. It is both subject and object. It is its own outlet and its own material. It is. All the rest of us are divided bits of self, some here, some there. The cat has a complete subjective unity. Being its own centre, it radiates electricity in all directions. It is magnetic and impervious. I have known people to keep a cat so they could stroke the electricity out of it. Why didn't they know how to be electric as the cat IS? The cat is the fine specimen of the I am. Who of us is so fully the I am that I am?

Look around the world! Everybody putting himself out in some form or another! Why? It doesn't do any good.

At the end you exhaust the possibilities of the outside world—geographically and spiritually. You can use up the external. You can come to the end of objectifying and objectives, and then what? In the end, only what we started with—the Self in the body, the Self at home, where it was all the time while bits of it were wandering outside.

Isn't it interesting how cats, who say nothing, are given so much to say by the people who attempt to govern them, their sometime friends? We humans love cats as metaphors more than animals it would seem. But, taken either way, they have their sway, and own us, never the reverse.

The Lore of the Cat

The gorgeous chrysanthemum of a cat known to the world as the white Persian is actually a descendant of the Turkish Angora. In Great Britain each color of Persian is considered a separate breed, but in the United States each one is believed to be a Persian of separate color. The only varieties of white Persian are cats with different colored eyes; they may be orange-eyed, blue-eyed, or odd-eyed. The fur is always thick and dense and it forms a leonine mane. The face is flat, the nose short, the head round. The ears are rounded at the tip and relatively small, with tufting inside.

The classic Persian body is broad and solid with short thick legs and large round paws. This is not known to be a particularly athletic cat, though there are many instances where Persians do extraordinary things, like the black Persian that could jump ten feet into the air and alight among the knickknacks of a lofty shelf.

Historically, the Persian was a temple cat, a companion of royalty, an emissary of souls passing from life to death. The heraldic Persian face made her the perfect cold-eyed complement of the mastermind villain Blofeld in the James Bond series. This cat's classic impassivity is there in that cloud of fur and stamped on the flattened face, the gimlet eyes, inscrutable and empty as the sky. Actually, the

Blofeld cat that appears in the film versions of *You Only Live Twice* and *Diamonds Are Forever* is a snowy white chinchilla whose appropriate biblical name is Solomon.

Of all the breeds, the Persian is still the most popular worldwide. Perhaps the cat's popularity comes from the Persian myth of King Hormus, who was told by a fortune-telling priest that his kingdom would one day be besieged. "You will have only twelve thousand men," the seer said, "but you will have to vanquish three hundred thousand enemies." The king begged to know how he might overcome the odds that were so heavily laid against him, and the seer answered, "You will have to find, somewhere in your kingdom, a man with the face of a cat." When the time came, the king did that thing—found the very man—and defeated the armies against him.

There is also the tale of the old Gaelic king who was, it's said, cat-headed. His name was Carbar, and in Ireland, to this day, tales are told of the cat armies that went out into the field and of warriors with strange wildcat skins on their helmets.

A fourteenth-century Persian myth sings the praises of the Persian cat hero in the great battle of the cats and the rats. Such a fight, by the way, is so universal that few countries do not have some version of it. The rodents, the story goes, have superior weaponry, but the felines have their natural defenses—claws, wits, and fangs. In the final battle, the hero cat is taken prisoner, and in one version of the tale, the rats, as a result of this maneuver, are victorious. In another version, however, the cat hero is greatly underestimated by the rat leader, who, having already taken him prisoner, merely ties him to a stake. With "the claws like an eagle and the tail of a serpent," the Persian cat hero bursts from his bonds and single-handedly routs all of the rats.

So it is that the cat and the rat (and let's not forget the dog!) are the most pervasive, universal fables we possess as a world culture, but of the cats, none figures more elegantly, more persistently, and more heroically than that gimlet-eyed mistress of the cloud realm, the artistic Persian.

THE ARCHETYPAL CAT

Tabby

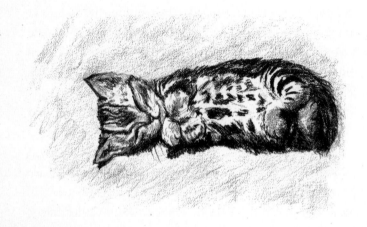

WILLIAM BLAKE HAD the archetypal cat in mind when he wrote the finest feline poem of all time, "The Tyger." The poem, like the cat that inspired it, is a series of unanswered, and largely unanswerable, questions. The illustrations done by the poet-artist are equally enigmatic. In some copies of the book, the tiger is a voracious beast, but in others it seems to be a tame pussycat. Perhaps it is, and always was, a little of each, a combination tiger and tabby.

Is it because the big cat chose not to lie down with the lamb that we consigned it to oblivion? Is it hovering there now, its fearful symmetry slowly fading in the forests of the night? Poet Halsey Davis, remembering his service years on the border of Burma and China during the Second World War, once recalled for us the night that a tiger, right out of Blake's imaginary mold, walked into his tent.

We were camped on that borderland near the airstrip, when the tiger came into our camp. We were sleeping, or we were supposed to be asleep, but on some nights I would lie awake listening to the singing frogs, or the rain falling, or some nights, just listening. I was listening when the tiger entered our tent.

It walked in, as pretty as you please—the grandest and most spectacular tiger you could ever imagine. The wooden floor of the tent platform creaked under its weight, as it padded from bed to bed, sniffing heads. I don't think anyone was awake but me. I lay in a pool of cold sweat, trying to subdue my heart. That tiger moved from bunk to bunk, examining and smelling each head, so circumspectly. It seemed to me a century before he finally came over and lowered his wide whiskered face, and brought it down level with mine.

I could smell his breath and it did not smell minty, I can assure you. The largeness of that head filled the space above my own in such a way that I felt warmer because of it. And it stayed there beside me for a good while, during which time the pool of sweat I lay in, filled the cavity made by my backside. I was chilled and overheated at the same time, an experience I shall never forget. At last, for no fathomable reason, the tiger left. As it turned to leave the tight quarters between bunks, its upcurved tail banged against my bed frame, and the solidity of it sent my heart skipping like a bird.

The last thing I remember, after daring myself to open my eyes, was that magnificent tiger standing in the triangular doorway of the barracks tent, surveying the peaceful, slumbering scene for the last time. The opaque moonlight was spread foggily behind that huge feline frame. The tiger stood motionless, not emboldened by the moon, but stilled by it. His head—and that is what I remember most after all these years—was as big as a boulder.

It sort of blotted out everything else, as the giant cat hesitated there, unmoving.

What was it doing? What was it thinking? I've asked myself that question many times, and never come up with a satisfactory answer. Then, the tiger rotated itself, stripes converging, and went out into the white Burmese night.

The human fascination with tigers, large and small, would seem, sometimes, to be reciprocal. Are we as interesting to them as they are to us? Do big cats have a philosophical, as well as culinary, interest in human beings? Domestic cats seem to find our investigations, our pastimes, our work and our rest, more interesting than we do. They, too, follow us, watching circumspectly, from afar. They measure our responses to things unknown to them and they grant us our private moments that other animals—dogs, for instance—do not grant as readily.

If only we were not so apt to confound one another. If only we knew one another better. If only we had the time and the wisdom to explore each of our fearful symmetries with unjudging love. And if only we might walk in and out of our respective domiciles, as the Burmese tiger did, curiously, silently, and without so much as a hint of harm.

Unfortunately, our access to large cats has always been too abrupt and too dangerous for our own good. Sadly, we've inspired their mistrust, their malicious playfulness, and we've mercilessly teased them under the big tent, the circus. We've caged them so we might consider them safely, but, in so doing, we've deprived them of their magnanimity. These things are certainly our undoing. Edward Hoagland in *The Courage of Turtles* speaks of the uneasy relationship between trainer and tiger:

First, he works alone with his cats, as lithe and on top of things as Clyde Beatty once was, but with a gentle, fertile, inventive delight, a sinful, delicious intimacy, and frank joy. . . . He gives them the "How" salute of an animal man

to a tiger, hand raised and palm flat, and bats them with
the butt end of his whip to keep them slinking and roaring,
nonplussed.

It's the nonplussed part that seems to have kept us from com-
munion with these great cats. That, and the "sinful, delicious, intimacy." And, on this, too, rides the plethora of hidden feelings
between the caged cat and the thinking human being. They, whether
caged or free are always locked into nature, looking out; while we,
fallen angels, are locked out, looking in. Our failure to communicate
doesn't hinge upon our mutual preference for pounds of meat, but
rather our intentional refusal to accept what William Blake called the
tiger's "fearful symmetry":

> *Tyger, Tyger, burning bright,*
> *In the forests of the night;*
> *What immortal hand or eye,*
> *Could frame thy fearful symmetry?*

We know the answer to this cat-striped, tabby-ticklish riddle.
But it's just as Halsey Davis said: "I don't have to ask what immortal
hand or eye could frame the fearful symmetry—I know, believe me,
I know."

And, in truth, so do we.

The Lore of the Cat

The tabby cat, while not a breed, but rather a color, has become over
the centuries a cultural icon. His progenitor, say some authorities, was
the Kaffir cat, a yellowish feline with tiger stripes, *Felis lybica,* which
still roams about northeastern Africa, hunting at night and living in
holes dug by other animals. Carl Van Vechten, author of *The Tiger in
the House,* states that "the Romans brought the Egyptian cat to England some time before the fifth century and there is a theory to the

effect that our modern tabby is a cross between this ancient animal and the British wild cat."

Jean Conger in *The Velvet Paw* suggests the earliest domesticated cat was the so-called tabby: "The pet of Pharaohs was a yellow cat with black stripes which became more distinct as they approached the tip of his tail. Ah! Here is a miniature tiger. So much do the old wall-paintings across the river from Memphis and Thebes tell us."

Other writers, like Frances and Richard Lockridge, say that the tabby was at home in Ireland as long ago as 500 B.C.E., which conforms to myths still circulated in that country.

However it may be, or have come about, the amber-coated, tigery tabby is favored for many reasons, not the least of which is the fact that this cat was adopted in northern and southern Europe as the archetypal hearth cat. The cats of the hearth were mousers, of course, and butter watchers. But they were also mystic animals, capable of all kinds of magic. In Ireland, they sent the snakes, which were pitched into the sea by Saint Patrick, back to land. Some say this kept the balance of nature; others commented that it made Ireland a trickier place to live. Actually, the mythological reference here is the old Egyptian cat/serpent motif, but that is another story. In Italy and other sunny climes, the tabby was a sun cat, a happy-as-the-house-is-home cat, but also the favored animal of—would you believe—lawyers, their patron saint, in fact. Balance again, perhaps?

In a recent *Cat Fancy* article entitled "What Color Is Your Cat?" Carolyn Osier discusses the tabby and clears up the cloudy idea that this cat is a breed apart. She says, among other things, that

> it is a common mistake to think of the tabby as a breed of cat, when in fact it is a pattern that can occur on any type of body or cat. Some cats have an overriding gene that suppresses the tabby pattern and only allows us to see the solid color. But sometimes we can glimpse a pattern anyway. Look at a solid black cat in bright sunlight and you may see faint black stripes. And very often we see "ghost" stripes on kittens of all colors.

She goes on to say that the most dominant of tabby patterns is seen in the Abyssinian. This is the cat, you remember, with the mascara lines around the eyes, which Egyptian women liked so much they imitated it—and we today do the same, don't we? "The most commonly seen tabby pattern," Osier explains, "is called the mackerel." She continues, defining the subtlety of this coloration:

> The tracings extend over the top of the head, widening into the shape of the royal Egyptian scarab. . . . They continue down the cat's back, in lines along the spine. At right angles to the spine lines are straight lines along the cat's sides, forming a fishbone—or mackerel—pattern. Cats can have black stripes on a lighter red background (brown tabby), blue stripes on an ivory background (blue tabby), red stripes on a lighter red background (red tabby), cream on a paler cream background (cream tabby), chocolate on ivory (chocolate tabby) or even lilac on white (lilac tabby).
>
> For additional drama we can change the pattern to classic, or blotched, with a bull's-eye on the sides and shoulders, or a spotted pattern, in which lines or bull's-eyes are broken into spots. Since these are recessive patterns we rarely see them in random-bred cats. Sometimes the tabby pattern appears over the tortoiseshell or blue-cream color so that parts of it appear in different color combinations. We describe these color combinations as patched tabby or torbie.

Regardless of what the tabby is, however, in terms of coloration, our oldest myths explain how this well-fed, easily domesticated, self-satisfied (Morris of 9-Lives) feline got to be what he is today—a couch potato. The rule is, he is doing what he was bred so long ago to do. The myth states that this cat once lived in the wild with a tiger. One day, when it was very cold, the tiger asked the tabby to please find him some extra warmth, and the tabby went off to find it. What he found was a human domicile, with a warm fire crinkling in the hearth. Sneaking in the window and stealing a firebrand, the tabby returned to the tiger and gave him his offering of fire, whereupon the tiger expressed his thanks. But now the tabby had a problem: his mind was full of that cheerful, firelit scene. The warm hearth beckoned, and he returned to it, a changed cat. In the end, he told the tiger, "I have found a better place, forgive me if I stay there forever."

And so he has.

Authors' Biography

GERALD AND LORETTA Hausman are authors of *The Mythology of Dogs: Canine Legend and Lore through the Ages* (St. Martin's Press, 1997). The Hausmans have been animal lovers and keepers of dogs and cats since the mid-sixties. Gerald Hausman's animal and Indian Lore books have been translated into six foreign languages and are also available on audio. *Meditations with Animals* was presented as a gift to high school teachers in Russia by the American antiarmament group STOP. Other new books by Mr. Hausman that feature animals are *Doctorbird: Three Lookin' Up Tales from Jamaica* (Philomel) and *The Story of Blue Elk* (Clarion). In 1995 Gerald Hausman was awarded the Aesop Accolade Award for *Duppy Talk: West Indian Tales of Mystery and Magic*. When not living in their home in Bokeelia, Florida, with their Great Dane, Zeb; dachshund, Beeper; Akita, Mocha; Siamese cat, Moonie; and blue-fronted Amazon, George, the Hausmans spend time traveling and learning more about the world of animals.

Bibliography

Altman, Roberta. *The Quintessential Cat*. New York: Macmillan, 1994.

Amory, Cleveland. *The Best Cat Ever*. Boston: Little, Brown, 1993.

————. *The Cat Who Came for Christmas*. New York: Penguin, 1988.

————. *The Cat and the Curmudgeon*. Boston: Little, Brown, 1990.

Basho. *The Narrow Road to the Deep North and Other Travel Sketches*. New York: Penguin, 1995.

Blake, William. *Songs of Innocence and of Experience*. New York: Oxford University Press, 1986.

Cameron, Angus, and Peter Parnall. *The Nightwatchers*. New York: Four Winds Press, 1971.

Caras, Roger A. *A Celebration of Cats*. New York: Simon and Schuster, 1986.

Caro, Frank de. *The Folktale Cat*. New York: Barnes and Noble, 1992.

Carroll, Lewis, and Martin Gardner. *The Annotated Alice*. Cleveland/New York: World, 1965.

Charters, Ann. *Kerouac: A Biography*. New York: Warner, 1974.

Cirlot, J. E. *A Dictionary of Symbols*. New York: Philosophical Library, 1962.

Conger, Jean. *The Velvet Paw: A History of Cats in Life, Mythology, and Art*. New York: Ivan Obolensky, 1963.

Corey, Paul. *Do Cats Think?* Chicago: Henry Regnery, 1977.

Dale-Green, Patricia. *Cult of the Cat*. Boston: Houghton Mifflin, 1963.

Duggan, Colm. *Treasures of Irish Folklore*. New York: Arlington House, 1983.

Gettings, Fred. *The Secret Lore of the Cat*. New York: Carol, 1989.

Gilbert, John R. *Cats, Cats, Cats, Cats*. London: Paul Hamlyn, 1961.

Graves, Robert. *The White Goddess*. New York: Farrar, Straus and Cudahy, 1948.

Greene, David. *Incredible Cats*. London: Methuen, 1984.

Grossman, Gary H., and Robb Weller. *A&E's Incredible World of Cats*. New York: A&E Home Video/New Video Group, 1996. Videocassette.

Gustafson, Ralph. *The Penguin Book of Canadian Verse*. New York: Penguin, 1958.

Hamilton, Elizabeth. *Cats: A Celebration*. New York: Scribners, 1979.

Hass, Robert. *The Essential Haiku: Versions of Basho, Buson, and Issa*. Hopewell, New Jersey: Ecco Press, 1994.

Hausman, Gerald. *Meditations with Animals*. Santa Fe: Bear and Company, 1986.

————. *Turtle Island Alphabet: A Lexicon of Native American Symbols and Culture*. New York: St. Martin's Press, 1992.

Hemingway, Ernest. *Islands in the Stream*. New York: Bantam, 1972.

Howey, M. Oldfield. *The Cat in Magic*. London: Bracken, 1993.

Irons, Glenwood. *Gender, Language, and Myth: Essays on Popular Narrative*. Toronto: University of Toronto Press, 1992.

Jarrell, Randal. *The Animal Family*. New York: Pantheon, 1965.

Joseph, Michael. *Cat's Company*. London: Hazell, Watson, and Viney, 1930.

Kerouac, Jack. *Big Sur*. New York: Bantam, 1962.

————. *Book of Dreams*. San Francisco: City Lights, 1961.

Kherdian, David. *Country Cat, City Cat*. New York: Four Winds Press, 1978.

————. *Threads of Light*. Aurora, Ore.: Two Rivers Press, 1985.

Khury, Samantha. *Samantha Khury: I Talk to Animals*. Produced and directed by Peter Friedman. New York: WLIW, 1991. Videocassette.

Kinsella, Thomas. *The New Oxford Book of English Verse*. New York: Oxford University Press, 1986.

Kirk, Mildred. *The Everlasting Cat*. Woodstock, N.Y.: Overlook Press, 1977.

Kuncl, Tom. *All about Cats*. Boca Raton, Fla.: Globe Communications, 1996.

Lahr, John. *Coward, the Playwright*. London: Methuen, 1982.

Lindskold, Jane M. "The Well-named Cat." 1997.

Lockridge, Richard and Frances. *Cats and People*. Philadelphia: Lippincott, 1950.

Masson, Jeffrey Moussaieff, and Susan McCarthy. *When Elephants Weep: The Emotional Lives of Animals*. New York: Delta, 1996.

Mery, Fernand. *The Life, History, and Magic of the Cat.* New York: Grosset and Dunlop, 1969.

Moyes, Patricia. *How to Talk to Your Cat.* New York: Wings, 1993.

Oates, Joyce Carol, and Daniel Halpern. *The Sophisticated Cat.* New York: Penguin, 1992.

Osier, Carolyn. "What Color Is Your Cat?" *Cat Fancy,* July 1997.

Pound, Ezra. *Selected Poems.* New York: New Directions, 1957.

Powell, James N. *The Tao of Symbols.* New York: Quill, 1982.

Repplier, Alice. *The Fireside Sphynx.* Boston/New York: Houghton Mifflin, 1901.

Rilke: Selected Poems. Translated by C. F. MacIntyre. Berkeley: University of California Press, 1962.

Ross, Lillian. *Portrait of Hemingway.* New York: Simon and Schuster, 1961.

Rutherford, Alice Philomena. *The Reader's Digest Illustrated Book of Cats.* Montreal, Canada: Reader's Digest, 1992.

Saroyan, William. *Here Comes, There Goes, You Know Who.* New York: Barricade, 1995.

———. *Tracy's Tiger.* New York: Ballantine, 1967.

Schneck, Marcus, and Jill Caravan. *Cat Facts.* New York: Barnes and Noble, 1990.

Service, William. *Owl.* New York: Knopf, 1969.

Siegal, Mordecai. *Simon and Schuster's Guide to Cats.* New York: Fireside, 1983.

Simmons, Eleanor Booth. *Cats.* New York: Whittlesey House, McGraw-Hill, 1935.

Simms, Katharine L. *They Walked Beside Me.* London: Hutchinson, 1955.

Spector, Norman B. *The Complete Fables of Jean de la Fontaine.* Evanston, Ill. Northwestern University Press, 1988.

Suares, Jean-Claude, and Seymour Chwast. *The Literary Cat.* New York: Berkley, 1977.

Taylor, Theodore. *The Cat.* New York: Avon, 1969.

Thomas, Elizabeth Marshall. *The Tribe of Tiger: Cats and Their Culture.* New York: Simon and Schuster Audioworks, 1994.

Twain, Mark. *The Unabridged Mark Twain.* Philadelphia: Running Press, 1979.

Van de Wettering, Janwillem. *The Empty Mirror: Experiences in a Japanese Zen Monastery.* Boston: Houghton Mifflin, 1974.

Van Vechten, Carl. *Peter Whiffle: His Life and Works*. New York: Knopf, 1923.

———. *The Tiger in the House*. New York: Dorset Press, 1989.

Warner, Sylvia Townsend. *The Cat's Cradle Book*. New York: Viking Press, 1940.

Williams, Joy. *The Florida Keys: A History and Guide*. New York: Random House, 1993.

Williams, Oscar. *A Little Treasury of Modern Poetry English and American*. New York: Scribners, 1952.

Williams, Tennessee. *One Arm and Other Stories*. New York: New Directions, 1954.

Winslow, Helen M. *Concerning Cats: My Own and Some Others*. New York: Lothrop, 1900.

Wylder, Joseph. *Psychic Pets: The Secret World of Animals*. New York: Stonehill, 1978.

Yeats, W. B. *The Celtic Twilight*. New York: New American Library, 1962.

Zelazny, Roger. *When Pussywillows Last in the Dooryard Bloomed*. Victoria, Australia: Norstrillia Press, 1980.

———. *To Spin Is Miracle Cat*. San Francisco: Underwood-Miller, 1981.

Index